Ribbons of Faith

Annette Courtney Ferrell

Copyright © 2011

ISBN: 978-0-9836648-7-1

Dust Jacket Press
PO Box 721243
Oklahoma City, OK 73172
www.dustjacket.com <http://www.dustjacket.com>
800-495-0192

Graphic Design: Lyn Rayn

To my husband, James, who means everything to me:
You are the most wonderful husband in the entire world! Our lives took an amazing turn that summer day and your strength, humor and steadfast presence have been a source of pure joy for me. You have been the supportive and loving husband every woman wants to have. This is quite a journey we are on and there is absolutely no one else with whom I would rather take it. I love you!

To my parents, Mike and Ruth Courtney:
Mom, I always wanted to grow up to be just like you, with your gentle and quiet spirit. You are a rock of strength and love that flows from your deep faith in the Lord. Your life has been an example of holy living that I want to emulate.

Dad, the years as a pastor refined your outstanding ability as a wordsmith and I am grateful some of it was passed along to me. I can even thank you for making me look up the definitions and spelling in the old Webster's Dictionary! Your prayers for me and your humorous stories have both been a source of great encouragement.

Contents

Introduction

We all have those dates on our calendar to remember a moment that took our breath away:

- high school graduation
- the birth of a child
- sunrise on a crystal clear day
- our wedding day
- being hired at the job we worked so hard to get
- hearing "I love you" for the first time
- moving into our dream home

And then there are moments that kick us in the stomach and knock the breath right out of us!

In June 2000, I was diagnosed with breast cancer. There was no history of breast cancer in my family, so this took me completely by surprise. During the eleven months from diagnosis to the final radiation treatment, I was on a journey like no other I have ever experienced.

Since that traumatic date I have sometimes worn a pink ribbon to mark myself as a breast cancer survivor. It seems now that there is an awareness ribbon for almost every kind of medical or social disorder. Almost everyone knows that pink is for breast cancer, but here are some other awareness ribbons:

- Red, for HIV/AIDS, heart disease, or pro-life
- Jigsaw or Puzzle, for Autism or Asperger Syndrome
- Orange, for self-injury awareness, ADHD, or leukemia
- Silver, for ovarian cancer, elderly abuse, or learning disabilities
- Black, for mourning, sleep disorders, or gun control
- Yellow, for support our troops, missing children, liver disease
- Purple, for lupus, Crohns disease, cystic fibrosis, or pancreatic cancer
- Green, for Lyme disease or organ transplantation

The list of awareness ribbons seems endless and almost all colors share various meanings, but the common theme is awareness. Wearing a ribbon says, "I want you to notice this disease/disorder/issue!"

This book is my story. While my story is a journey through breast cancer, the theme is not so much "cancer" as it is "faith." And it was faith in God through a relationship with Jesus Christ that was my anchor through all the ups and downs of this part of my life. This book is not a comprehensive medical or theological discourse. It was born out of the journal entries I made during the first year after the diagnosis. Underneath it all is a confidence in the Living God who I was sure would bring me through "not somehow, but triumphantly." That is the title of a devotional book by Dr. Bertha Munro and seems to best describe my attitude. I didn't know if I would survive, but I knew where my hope came from.

Cancer is a terrifying disease. Enduring the treatments took everything I could muster—and then some. It has been eleven years since the diagnosis and, while there have been additional scares along the way, as of this writing, I am cancer free.

Whatever the color of awareness ribbon you may wear—whether you or a loved one is dealing with a physical disease, emotional turmoil, or any other challenge life throws at you—this book is written with the hope that it will be an encouragement to you. We can wear our awareness ribbons and let them be ribbons of faith.

Acknowledgments

There is a host of individuals who helped make this book possible. It seems that a simple "thank you" is not enough, but it is all I have to give. My deepest gratitude is extended to you who have shown me kindnesses over and over!

Pastor Jim Williams of Lake View Park Church of the Nazarene, who gave wise counsel to me and my husband in the early days, when cancer was still only a possibility. Your spiritual leadership and friendship continues to be a blessing to us. I remember my surprise when you said, "You ought to write a book." I had no idea what would be worth saying, but you planted an idea and God has brought it to this point.

My friend, Beta Noel, gave me the courage to believe that James' selection of a red wig was the best choice when my hair fell out. A few years later, as we sat in the restaurant and I told you I was trying to write a book, you encouraged me with your immediate support, helping me to believe that I could do it. Your expertise with the English language has been a priceless asset to me.

Not too many people in the world will adjust their own schedule to help a friend in need, but Nona-Sue Mellish and Tami Waits did just that! You gave your time at my bedside when I needed extra care. You were truly God's hands and feet as chauffeurs and aides, serving in many ways.

The entire congregation of Lake View Park Church of the Nazarene in Oklahoma City gathered around us in a loving circle of practical help and spiritual support. James and I could not have survived without your incredible acts of kindness.

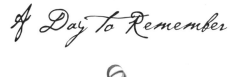

ONE

"Annette, I have to be honest with you. *This looks really ugly; it is probably cancer. I don't want to scare you, but you need to be prepared when you come back on Thursday for the results.*"

This was the statement from the doctor who was just finishing the needle biopsy on my left breast. His words literally took my breath away. I was surprised that I could even dress and walk out of the room.

How could this be happening? What was going to come next? Could it really only be five days since all this started?

The morning of June 15, 2000, dawned like any other workday. My husband of nineteen years, James, arose early and left the house for his job as a framing carpenter. His crew was working in a housing addition in a growing suburb of Oklahoma City.

I had taken the day off for a couple of appointments, so I was enjoying a slower start. While in the shower, our house phone rang once, then twice, then again and again. I yelled out in frustration that I'd be there in a minute. No one heard me but our cat. Caller ID told me it was James, so I quickly dialed his cell phone.

"I fell off a ladder. I think I broke my ankle. I need you to come take me to the doctor," James barely spoke through the pain. He told me he had made it to a friend's house close to his work site. I threw on some clothes and made my way out to our friend's home, praying all the way that he would be okay.

Upon arriving at their home, I found James lying on their newly tiled kitchen floor. He was glad for the cool surface since the increasing pain was making him nauseous. Thankfully, Tami had been home that morning and graciously allowed James to literally collapse on their floor. At 8:30 I called our family doctor's office and they agreed to work him in quickly. Tami helped me get James to the car, even giving us some plastic trash bags, in case he threw up on the way. The pain was so intense that he could barely talk. Every expansion joint in the road was like torture to his body.

An x-ray and exam by our family doctor confirmed the worst: a severe sprain to the right ankle. The swelling was already so pronounced that they couldn't see where the break was, though the doctor was sure the bone was broken. They set James' ankle in a "half cast" of wet plaster strips held in place with Ace bandages, to immobilize the joint while waiting for the swelling to subside. Armed with a prescription for pain medication, I took James home. Once inside, he fell into the recliner and I prepared a simple lunch, which he didn't eat.

While waiting at the doctor's office, I had cancelled my hair appointment that was scheduled for late morning. I felt I should keep my annual exam with the gynecologist, so after lunch I washed my hair and dressed for the afternoon. About two weeks earlier, I had noticed a lump near the surface of my left breast. Since it was about time for my annual exam, I decided to wait and have it checked at that time. It had appeared suddenly and I was more curious than concerned. I guessed it was a cyst that could be drained or removed without trouble.

The doctor was unavailable, but a very capable Physician's Assistant took care of the routine exam. She was very concerned about the lump and asked questions: When was my last mammogram? Was there a history of breast cancer in my family? How long had the lump been there? Had there been any redness or soreness? That was when I first realized it wasn't a cyst after all, but the word "cancer" was still not in my mind. She went to the phone to get me an immediate appointment at a nearby facility for a mammogram.

When they were finally able to work me in, the technician had to manually enter the settings because my breast tissue is extremely dense and the pre-programmed settings weren't reading well. As soon as that was finished, I waited again for an ultrasound on the left breast. No one said the word "cancer" but the longer I waited, the more uptight I became and slowly realized this was much more serious than I first expected.

Friday morning I returned to work as the secretary for my church. Had it not been the busiest day of the week for me, I would have taken off a second day to care for James. At about ten o'clock my gynecologist called to tell me that the doctor at the Breast Care Center was "very concerned" about the lump, because of its size and density. They scheduled me for a biopsy the following Tuesday morning.

I thought I could keep my focus at work, but suddenly I felt like I would fall apart. I asked my pastor, Jim Williams, if I could talk to him for a few minutes. As I explained what had happened and the phone call I just received, he was very understanding and realized that I was on edge. He suggested that I close the office and go home. After all, James still needed some extra attention. Jim also told me that his sister had breast cancer years ago and he understood a little of what I was feeling.

A group of people was meeting at the church office, so after they left and it was quiet, I tried to work but found I could not focus at all. I found myself with hands poised over the keyboard, but lost in thought. I decided to follow my Pastor's advice and go home. I told James about the doctor's call, trying of course, to keep my thoughts from racing ahead to disaster. Mostly, I fidgeted around the house, unable to concentrate on anything. James was really nauseated all that morning and finally threw up around noon. He said he actually felt a whole lot better after that. We figured it was the medicine, so he started eating before taking a pill.

Pastor Jim came by the house later that afternoon to check on us. As we talked, I expressed my reluctance to say anything "public" just yet about this lump and upcoming biopsy. Both James and Pastor suggested I tell a few close friends and ask them to be praying for me ... after all, that's part of what the church is for. No need to be strong and quiet when prayer support can help turn the focus from what might be to the truth of who God is.

Saturday afternoon we attended a wedding. We arrived early to get a back-row seat so James could keep his leg elevated while staying out of the way. After the wedding I was able to speak to a couple of friends, telling them what was happening. One of them asked if I would meet her at the altar for prayer at church on Sunday.

In our church we have an "open altar," which means that, at the appointed time, anyone can go kneel for prayer for any reason. That Sunday morning, James was unable to walk to the front with me but several friends met me there to pray for me. When faced with catastrophic news, it is so good to know you're not alone!! It was very hard for me to pray. Emotions and fear kept my mind racing. I was only able to say a simple prayer over and over, "Jesus, help me."

On Monday evening I was reading some scripture, really searching for a promise from God that He would heal me and spare me from cancer. I didn't find anything like that. Instead, I found these words:

Matthew 11:28-30: "Come to me, all you who are weary and burdened, and I will give you rest. Take my yoke upon you and learn from me, for I am gentle and humble in heart, and you will find rest for your souls. For my yoke is easy and my burden is light."

Matthew 6:25-27, 33: "Therefore, I tell you, do not worry about your life, what you will eat or drink; or about your body, what you will wear. Is not life more important than food, and the body more important than clothes? Look at the birds of the air; they do not sow or reap or store away in barns, and yet your heavenly Father feeds them. Are you not much more valuable than they? Who of you by worrying can add a single hour to his life? And why do you worry about clothes? But seek first his kingdom and his righteousness and all these things will be given to you as well."

As I began to look to God for strength, instead of looking inward at my own fear, I was able to accept that there might not be healing in my immediate future. I came to a place where I could honestly say, "Lord, not my will, but yours."

Tuesday morning came and the biopsy was done. After the doctor told me it was probably cancer, I drove us home. Though unable to drive, James was adamant about being there with me. When we got to our driveway, I didn't need to control my emotions any longer, so through the tears, I told him what the doctor said. It was very hard to even say the word "cancer."

My parents had also been there during the biopsy. Once we all were seated in our living room, I told them what the doctor had said. We talked for just a few minutes, speculating about the advances in treatment for breast cancer. Then my parents went home. I think they were shocked as much as we were. My father is a retired pastor and never lacks for something to say, but that day he was very subdued. James and I talked for a while, trying to make a little sense of it all. Mostly, I just cried. I called Pastor Jim and told him that I wouldn't be in the office the rest of the day and gave him the news as well.

It was emotionally draining to ponder what might be ahead. During the day I could imitate Scarlett O'Hara from "Gone with the Wind" and say, "Fiddle-dee-dee, I'll think about it tomorrow." At night, though, when all was quiet, the tears flowed.

The pathology report came back in two days: Stage 2 Moderately Differentiated Infiltrating Ductal Carcinoma. It sounded positively terrifying. James and I received an inch-thick packet of information and were told, "don't try to read it all at once—there's too much detail here." (I tried anyway and they were right.) The tumor was 5 centimeters (about 2 inches) and had two small satellite tumors near the lymph nodes ... but appeared not to have invaded the lymph system. A mastectomy was the prescribed treatment, followed by both chemotherapy and radiation. The entry from my journal that day reads:

"We went home and just cried together. I know I'm a control freak—can't deny that—and this kind of thing is really hard to accept. From books I've read, I know my whole life is about to change dramatically. I've never liked sudden change and this scares me. All I can think of is, 'I don't want to do this. Oh, God, help me. I want to be healed and not go through a bunch of junk. I don't like pain; uncertainty scares me.' But then I recall part of a song I heard recently on the radio, 'I will go through the valley if you want me to.'"

I have called myself a Christian all of my life. My father was a pastor in the Church of the Nazarene, so I was raised in the church. My mother is a godly woman whose gentle, quiet spirit has been my example. I attended a university whose motto is Character, Culture, Christ. James and I had been through tumultuous times before in our marriage—the frustrations of infertility, the deep despair of losing two children during pregnancy, financial setbacks. However, in everything, God has always been trustworthy and provided what we needed to make it through to better days.

This time, though, it was my very life. How would I deal with it all? *Could* I deal with it? I eventually found out that what I heard in a sermon is true: "We are like coffee cups and when we get bumped around by life, what's inside is what sloshes over the edge."

On Sunday morning after the biopsy, following a very emotional week where I tried to work but mostly went through the motions, my pastor preached a sermon from the 73rd Psalm. The chapter begins with these words:

"Surely God is good to Israel, to those who are pure in heart. But as for me, my feet had almost slipped; I had nearly lost my foothold. For I envied the arrogant when I saw the prosperity of the wicked. They have no struggles; their bodies are healthy and strong. They are free from the burdens that come to man...

"When I tried to understand all this, it was oppressive to me till I entered the sanctuary of God, then I understood their final destiny.

"My flesh and my heart may fail, but God is the strength of my heart and my portion forever."

Of course the pastor immediately had my attention! Not only did I feel that I had been going down a slippery slope all week, I had crashed at the bottom of the hill and was in a terrible state. All around me there were healthy people going about their daily business, with no regard to the turmoil I was in. Was it true, this faith in God that I professed? Why did God let this happen? Why wouldn't He just take it away? What would happen to me? Would I die quickly? Would I go through months of treatment and then die anyway?

My husband is the sound technician at our church and I sit with him at the back of the sanctuary. It is not unusual for me to be distracted during any given service by things that happen between the front and the back. However, when Pastor Jim preached that day, it seemed as though he was standing right in front of me, speaking directly to me. In reality, I knew that there were many people in my extended church family who were hurting along with me or even had their own unwanted circumstances to deal with. As Pastor Jim preached words of truth and encouragement, my thinking was again directed to the truth of who God is.

There are times in every life when we have important spiritual decisions to make. That Sunday morning was a turning point for me. I made the choice, again, to believe that what I had learned about God all my life and experienced first-hand, was true. He is a God of love and compassion and cared deeply for me, regardless of the circumstances thrown at me. He was not a distant god with closed ears. He was (and is) a living God whose hands were strong enough to carry me through the hardest days of my life.

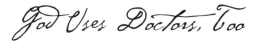

TWO

One week had passed since the diagnosis. Our family physician, Dr. Barry Mitchell, had begun to refer me to various other doctors for specialized care. The hardest part was waiting for the appointments. The doctors he preferred were out of town when first called, then there was the July 4th holiday weekend, both of which served to make it seem like nothing was happening. In the meantime, I read and re-read the information on breast cancer. I figured that by the time I saw an oncologist I would at least be familiar with the terminology.

In the course of one of James' follow-up appointments, Dr. Mitchell asked me if I had heard from the surgeon's office. He looked surprised when I said I had not. Then I was the one surprised when he walked out of the room, took a few steps to his own office and called his colleague. I could hear the conversation and it was only a couple of minutes when he came back with an appointment time on a slip of paper. At that moment, I could see how much he cared about us as persons, not just patients. He had paid attention when I told him the waiting was terrible.

James and I were finding a new routine to our days, which included appointments with doctors and calls from friends. It was during this time that I discovered how truly amazing e-mail could be. Since 1989 I have been the Office Administrator for Lake View Park Church of the Nazarene in Oklahoma City. Longevity in such a workplace begets some privileges and blessings, one of which is a vast network of people who wanted to know how I was doing. The following e-mail provides a glimpse into what became a regular way of communication.

Thursday, 6 July

Hello, all. It's Thursday evening and there has been quite a bit going on the last couple of days. Hope you don't mind a detailed update. Thanks for continuing to pray for us. I so strongly believe God is going ahead of us, giving wisdom, and helping in ways we don't even know yet.

First, James is improving a lot! Yesterday, he was able to take a few steps and put some weight on his foot. He was so excited!! Today he drove (carefully) out to where his crew is working ... made it back successfully. There was swelling in his foot while he moved around, so he spent the afternoon in the recliner. But, there is definite improvement and he is pleased. Of course, the down side is that he is beginning to fidget — feeling good enough to move around some, but not good enough to be at work to spur his guys on to accomplish what needs to be done. He returns to the orthopedic doctor next Friday.

Wednesday afternoon, James and I met with an oncologist, Dr. Charles Hollen. I believe it was a God-ordained meeting. He is very personable and spent about 45 minutes with us, answering questions, asking a few of his own, getting acquainted and beginning a relationship that will last a while. I was so impressed that he was not bothered by my long typed list of questions and did not talk down to us in highly technical terms no one could understand. He will be the "point doctor" in this adventure, the one to whom I'll address all my questions.

We reached the decision to have two doses of chemotherapy, then surgery. Next Tuesday morning, I'll go in for the first round of chemo. They'll hook me to an I.V. line and drip Adriamycin and Cytoxan (AC) for a couple of hours, make sure I'm okay, then send me home. In three weeks, I'll go for a second treatment. Three weeks after that, surgery, followed by more chemo after about 3-4 weeks recovery time. Total time involved is about 4-5 months. Then the decision will be made about radiation treatment.

So, we begin. Who knows how I'll feel this time next week! I'm glad we have a cordless phone so when friends call, I don't have to get off the couch! Pastor Jim has given me my "orders" that I am to be in the office only when I feel like it, so I'll try to behave and obey my boss! Really, though, I plan to continue normal activities as much as possible. When you see me out, you'll know I feel like being out.

You have been wonderfully supportive of me the last three weeks, and I am grateful for the cards, calls, and all the "little things" people have done. I do have one special request that would be enormously helpful: If you want to visit about how I'm doing, please call me at home. I'm having a hard time getting very much "real" work done at the office. Especially in the upcoming weeks, when at the office, I would like to be able to concentrate on the business of the church ... and take a break from thinking about myself. I hope you understand. A general "how are you" is quite all right, but I would prefer to keep that part of our conversations to a minimum. Of course, any other time I might just talk your ear off and tell you more than you ever wanted to know! Thanks for caring so much.

That's how we're doing. You all are wonderful friends and we are blessed beyond words to have you praying for us and loving us in many practical and amazing ways. We love you.

The first time we met with Dr. Hollen was quite memorable. James and I were waiting in the exam room. I had a typed list of questions in hand. James was seated, with his walking boot on and crutches at his side. The door opened and Dr. Hollen stepped inside, looked at James, then me, then back to James and asked, "What did she do to you?" As we laughed out loud, my first thought was, "A doctor with a sense of humor! I love it!" That was the beginning of a warm relationship between us and Dr. Hollen and his entire staff.

During that first appointment Dr. Hollen and his assistant covered in great detail the suggested treatments for breast cancer. Thanks to the packet given to me from the Breast Care Center, I was armed with two pages of questions, most of which I would never have thought of on my own. Some of those questions were:

- What kind of treatment will I receive? (chemotherapy, hormonal, immunotherapy)
- How often?
- How long will I receive treatments?
- What are the names of the drugs?
- What side effects will I experience? (nausea, hair loss, changes in blood cell counts, etc.)
- How will you evaluate the effectiveness of the treatments?
- Can I continue my usual work schedule?

A suggestion from one of the many "how to deal with cancer" booklets I read was to always have another person go to appointments with the patient. Most of the time, my husband was that extra set of eyes and ears. In any given appointment, I could zero in on one thing a doctor said and forget to listen to the rest of the conversation. That's how the brain sometimes responds when overloaded with details. At least, that's how MY brain works!

We fully discussed the various treatment options: chemotherapy, surgery, and radiation. It actually felt good to be proactive! For the first time in three weeks I felt like I could DO something, not have to wait for something to be done to me! Near the end of our first conversation with Dr. Hollen, James asked him, "If this was your wife, what would you advise her to do?" He said he would want her to receive the same treatment he was recommending. The response was honest and gave us something to consider as we made decisions.

One thing I learned during our conversation was that it was becoming more customary, though not standard treatment at that time, to begin chemotherapy before surgery. Dr. Hollen's opinion was that it would be the best way to see if "this tumor in this body responds well to this treatment"—and the only way to know that for sure would be to start chemotherapy before the tumor was removed. As I heard that, it made sense. James and I left for home with much to think and pray about. It was overwhelming, but we were at last able to begin fighting this thing called cancer.

A few days later I had my first cycle of chemotherapy. For those who have never been around someone who has received chemotherapy (as I had not been), here is how it all begins. This is part of an e-mail I sent out to friends and family members:

The treatment room is very large with big leather recliners around the perimeter, each with its own I.V. station, ready for a patient. It's a very casual atmosphere so that friends and family are welcome to come in—two at a time—to keep the patient company. They had soup mixes, crackers, soft drinks, etc. so that if the patient gets hungry, there's something to eat to help avoid nausea.

First, I gave two vials of blood for various tests. What they really want to know is if you're healthy enough to give you some poison! After I was given the go-ahead, they started the I.V. with a simple saline solution, the medium into which the other medicines were delivered. I bruised only a tiny bit, even on my fair skin. (Many patients choose to have a port surgically inserted under the skin of the upper chest wall. I decided to forgo the port, something I regretted later as the veins were harder to stick.)

Next was a dose of pre-medicines to fight nausea (Anzemet and Decadron), then the 100 mg of Adriamycin, which is a red liquid "pushed" from syringes, as opposed to dripping through an I.V.. Then, they gave me 1100 mg of Cytoxan, which took about an hour to drip. The entire procedure took about two and a half hours. My nurse was careful to make sure I understood everything, asking me how I felt and answering any questions. James was at my side the entire time.

The most immediate side effect of the drugs was a terrible sinus headache, which is a direct result of the Cytoxan. It went away sometime during the night, but left me pretty well wiped out on Wednesday morning, so I took my boss' advice and stayed home from work. Thankfully, there were volunteers who covered the office for me those two days, so I didn't feel any pressure to rush back to work.

The anti-nausea pills really worked, though I had some trouble on the third day after chemotherapy. I worked in the morning, but felt it was wise to go home at noon and get some rest. As far as food was concerned, I discovered that what sounded delicious one minute was quite revolting very shortly! A few nibbles here and there every hour weren't enough in the long run to keep me going so I was frequently frustrated while trying to figure out my new taste in foods.

There are several standard medications used to fight nausea caused by chemotherapy. Ativan, Phenergan, and Compazine have been around many years. When I started chemo, there was a fairly new "designer drug" on the market called Kytril. It was designed to turn off the part of the brain that receives the signal from the stomach that something needs to be thrown out. I took one the day of chemo, and the next two days. Since it was new, there was no generic available, and the cost at that time was $100 per pill. That alone is enough to make you nauseated! Thankfully, Kytril was on the approved list of medications, so it was covered by insurance.

I have a friend who had breast cancer in the 1970s. To this day, she can vividly remember the smells from the treatment room and the violent sickness she endured. I am so grateful that there are better options today.

The first cycle of chemotherapy was not as bad as I thought it would be. The level of care I received from my oncologist and nurses was excellent, which put me at ease.

Three days after the first chemo treatment, my husband and I attended a church staff planning retreat. It was an overnight event at a conference center outside of Norman, Oklahoma. Pastor Jim had asked each staff member to be prepared to share their goals for the next twelve months. My list was fairly short, but included one very specific goal: Surviving Cancer.

Years ago I heard about a book entitled "Not Somehow, But Triumphantly." I never got around to reading the book by Dr. Bertha Munro, but I loved the title and remembered it in the early days of cancer treatments. I determined in my mind and heart that if I had to go through such an awful thing, my personal goal would be to triumphantly survive. No eeking out a daily existence for me! Sometimes I could feel my inner child coming out. You've seen that child before ... the one who stomps her foot, crosses her arms, sticks out her lower lip and yells, "No!" Well, I was yelling "no!" to the thought of my life being consumed by cancer and its treatments. There was no getting around this, but I rebelled against the idea of it swallowing me up in its torrent.

During this time, I continued to read various scripture portions, allowing God's Word to encourage me. Deep down I really wanted to find a verse promising that my physical healing was right around the corner. Alas, that was not to be. Every time, and I do mean *every* time I picked up my Bible, I would run into more and more scriptures that talked about trusting God, holding on when the future looks bleak, resting on the promise of His love. One of my journal entries said:

I was looking at a calendar yesterday. If everything stays on the 3-week schedule, I should have my last chemo treatment right after Christmas. What a way to spend half a year. This is really working a number on my independent self: having to think about what to have around to eat to please my untrustworthy taste buds; having people constantly asking how I'm doing (and feeling like I should give them an answer); making sure I have my treatment and lab appointments written down—without fail; not being able to take aspirin that would knock out my headache!

Sounds like whining to me, but this is how I feel today. It's just the pits. I really would like God to miraculously heal me and be done with all this mess. But, I don't think

that's how God works—healing people for their own con-
venience. God does know my heart, though, and no matter
how I feel, He doesn't mind listening to my venting.

I believe in divine healing directly from God's hand. I also know that God uses doctors, too. It is nothing less than a divine miracle that doctors and researchers have created medical regimens to treat diseases. It is a miracle that prolongs life and defeats disease. While I prayed for God's instant healing touch, I had reached a place of trust in his human co-laborers and was ready for the fight.

THREE

Bald Is Beautiful
(Maybe)

I have always considered shopping for clothes and shoes a necessary evil, not the fun experience I hear about from other women. I enjoy looking good but hate spending the time and energy it takes to find those bargains. However, my hair is another story. I don't mind spending money on cuts, color or whatever is necessary in the attempt to get the look I want. I never thought much about how my hair defines who I am—or at the very least, what I think about myself. Even on bad hair days, at least it was my own hair.

Hair loss during chemotherapy is scary, in part because it is so public. There's just no hiding the fact that things are not normal. It is easy to be intimidated because people are curious and can't help but stare if a woman is bald.

It took only two weeks for my hair to start falling out. My oncologist told me to be prepared, but I was hoping to defy the odds. A few days after the first cycle of chemotherapy, my scalp started to hurt and tingle. Then I remembered the nurse telling me that would be the signal for the departure of my hair. Later, people would ask what it felt like and the best description I can give is this: It's like being outside on a windy day or taking a ride in a convertible. The wind through your hair is a great feeling ... until you have to comb out the tangles. That pulling and tugging feeling is similar to the sensation of hair loss from chemotherapy.

Wednesday, 26 July

More hair coming out—fast, now. When I styled my hair this morning, I had to stop and clear the strands from my brush. I don't want to do this. It hurts!!!!!!! Not physically, but I feel like I'm being taken apart, little by little. Friday afternoon is "D-day" when I pick up my wig. I don't want to go get my hair cut off and start wearing a wig. But even more, I don't want to wait too long and get up one morning to find I'm half bald with no "plan B" ready. Tonight James asked how I was doing and then the tears started. This is so hard! It was sweet of him to just hold me close and let me cry.

Thursday, 27 July

Oh, man, the fall-out continues. I've decided that the new definition of "mental anguish" is when you see your own hair filling up the sink when trying to blow dry. I am shedding everywhere. My stress level has gone up this week. I haven't checked my blood pressure, but it wouldn't surprise me if it were elevated.

Saturday, 29 July

James is sooooooooo good for me! Thursday night after we got in bed, I asked him if he wanted to run his hands through my hair "one last time" before I get sheared. He looked me straight in the eyes and said, "I already did when I picked up your hair from the bathroom floor." We laughed together, something I really needed. He also suggested that it might be hard for me to have a pity-party with him around.

Well, it's a done deal. My scalp is shaved and I have the wig. Beta Noel met us at the Boutique to help me decide which one I wanted. James and I had previously chosen a red wig, which is very different from my own color and I wanted another woman's perspective. I had a fright when the saleswoman couldn't find the wig immediately, but it only took her a couple of minutes to remember where she had stored it. Then we got down to business. It helped that Beta loved the color from the get-go. I went outside to look at the color again, making sure it didn't look orange in natural light.

James wanted me to be free to choose anything I wanted, even though he had suggested the red one, so I tried on another one that was shorter, blonde with a frosted look. Yuk! It made me look old with a sickly complexion. I sure don't need anything else making me appear even more pale and fragile! After making my decision, I asked the assistant to go ahead and cut my hair since I didn't want to do that at home.

As soon as she reached for the drape to keep the hair off my clothes, I started crying. She took the time to give me a little pep talk about how doing this now was part of taking control over the cancer ... not keeping to its time schedule, but creating my own. Sounded corny, but it's the truth, and her pep talk gave me enough time to settle my nerves and be fully prepared.

I let James take a picture of me after Darlene had finished with the electric shears. Forget vanity here, I want a record of this traumatic event! Then she reached for the shaver and went over a few spots to make sure the wig would conceal my hairline. Can you say "G.I. Jane"? After some trimming of the bangs and a snip here and there, she was finished shaping the wig to my face.

There were many thoughts rushing through my head as we left the Boutique: "Whew, that's over. Why are people looking at me? Can they tell it's a wig? Is it crooked and I can't feel it? Does it look so fake that people are smirking? Why do I care what strangers think, anyway?" (You'll notice all these were negative feelings. It took several days for me to really be comfortable with my new look.)

My parents were the first family members to see my new look. I think they were more than a little surprised at the color, but both agreed that it looked nice. James and I went to our church that evening for me to take pictures at Vacation Bible School. I felt like that would be the real test — seeing people I know and watching their reactions. Thankfully, there was much affirmation, which is what I needed. Some of the kids had questions about why I changed my hair, which gave me an opportunity to explain that I was taking some very strong medicine that caused my hair to fall out so the wig would be my hair for a while. In a funny way, their acceptance of it as fact without emotion did a lot to help me calm down.

Since my scalp was still very tender, I decided to go "natural" around the house. When my ears or scalp got chilled I donned one of the colorful turbans I had purchased. Though it was the middle of the summer, I was surprised at how cold I felt with my scalp uncovered. At night it actually helped me to sleep better to have something on my head. My scalp was too sensitive, plus I didn't want to have the pillowcase covered with little hairs every morning!

I ventured out on my own for a few errands the day after being fitted with the wig. The feelings of being watched, of thinking that people knew that it was not my own hair, were pretty strong. When I realized I was avoiding eye contact, I concentrated more on looking people in the eyes, just like I always have. It was tough, but I made it. When I got back home, I was exhausted!

Later that day, I found myself crying at anything. More of the grieving process, I suppose—that letting go of "what has been" and accepting the "what is now" in my life.

Within a few weeks I was very comfortable with my new look. I suppose it helped when strangers in elevators would compliment me on my hair. Somehow, I felt it was just fine that I was not obligated to explain that "my" hair was a wig because my "real" hair fell out during chemotherapy. After all, I paid good money for the wig – it really was mine!

FOUR

It Was Worse Than We Thought

Tuesday, 1 August

   Today is my 43rd birthday and has been a really good day in many ways. I feel pretty good, though off to a slow start this morning. Spent the day at work until about 4:00, then came home to rest.

   The staff had a little party during staff meeting—cake, ice cream, and a gift certificate to Foley's. Oooo, how nice! Then they took me to Steak & Ale for lunch. I am so spoiled by the staff it's ridiculous. But then again, I'm worth it! Ha! Ha!

   James and I have just returned from all-you-can-eat ribs at the Rib Crib. Found that they have that every Tuesday night, so we decided to check it out. It was very good! Of *course, it only took me 2 ribs, some onion rings and okra to be full, but James made up for it. Now he is praying for God to forgive him for being such a glutton. Ha!*

Had my second round of chemo yesterday, prefaced by another visit with Dr. Hollen. He was very pleased about my blood count—everything had rebuilt very well. He asked if I had any problems such as swelling in my feet or hands, or any other questions about overall health. The only thing I really asked him about was the severe arm pain from Saturday. He said there were two possible explanations: (1) That the steroid in the chemotherapy had worn off and there was a spike in inflammation in the joints; or (2) That the bone marrow was rebuilding and causing some expansion in the joints, which can be painful. He said he suspected option two, but that type of pain usually centered around the hips and pelvic area, simply because that is the highest concentration of bone mass in the body. Overall, he was very pleased by my outlook and general health.

We also talked about surgery date. He is connecting with the surgeon's office to schedule another appointment there before surgery, which will probably be around August 21 or 22. I've grown accustomed to the idea of a mastectomy, though I still don't like it. It's very scary to think about cutting off a part of my body, with all the attending recuperation and eventual reconstructive surgery. The few minor surgeries I have had pale in comparison to what this means. Sometimes I am overwhelmed with fear.

After the exam, I headed off for the treatment room. Mama was with me and we found the only remaining chair in the room. It was another 20 minutes or so before a nurse was free to hook me up and get things going. Not a bad thing; it's a comfortable place to wait. My dad and brother were running errands, including picking up my Kytril at the pharmacy.

Everything went well with chemo, though it just took longer. I wasn't finished until about 4:45. We got home around 5:00, just before Bill and Robbie arrived with supper. It was very good, but I didn't try the chicken. I'm sure it was great—James said so—but there was an aroma that didn't set too well in my nose. But I enjoyed the noodles, pears, cauliflower, and biscuit. Later I'll try the chocolate pie.

As the evening wore on, I was very fatigued and a little nauseated, so I took a Compazine pill. It helped settle my stomach, but then I felt really emotional. As we got into bed, it all came to a head and I cried on James' shoulder for a while. Sometimes it seems so overwhelming—all that is happening—and then the best way I know to deal with the emotion is to cry. I would love for this to be a nightmare and I'll wake up and everything would be "normal." But this is real life and it's going to be a long time before I see "normal" again.

Yesterday as I was waiting for Dr. Hollen, the old hymn came to my mind:

What have I to dread, what have I to fear?
Leaning on the everlasting arms.
I have blessed peace with my Lord so near.
Leaning on the everlasting arms.

It's true. There is so much going on inside of me—fear, insecurity, fatigue, occasionally times of utter hopelessness. Then there's also joy, resolve, hope for hard times to get better. When I remember Whose I am and Who holds me in His hands, I really do have that blessed peace the song describes. This is a tough journey, but I am not alone!

Tuesday, 15 August—e-mail to friends

Hello, everyone. It's time for another installment of "How the Ferrells Are."

This afternoon, James and I met with the surgeon to consult again before my surgery. (By the way, surgery is scheduled for 8:00 a.m. on Monday, August 21, at Deaconess Hospital.) I had my long list of questions ready and we started at the top: Has the chemotherapy shrunk the tumor? The answer is yes, so that's good news. That's one of the reasons I elected to have some chemo first, so it helps me to know it is having the desired effect on the tumor. However, it has not shrunk enough to leave any options for surgery. The surgeon will do a modified mastectomy. If you want details about what all that surgery entails, you can look it up on the web. I'll be in the hospital for a couple of days. He expects recovery at home to be anywhere from three to six weeks.

So, this week will be full of taking care of my "to do" list ... you know, all those things you put off doing until you're about to be out of town on vacation, or until you know the house guests are on the way to your front door. I promise—if I need help this week, I'll ask. :-)

I know you're all asking, "So, Annette, how are you REALLY doing?" Answer: There have been a few weeks to get accustomed to the idea of a mastectomy. I don't want it. Period. However, this seems to be the path for me right now and I am daily submitting my will to God's. Sometimes it's a struggle. But He knows my heart and I know He is stronger and wiser than I could ever be, so it's not a lengthy struggle. In His arms is a good place to be. James and I have had some very open discussions about our feelings about all this. The nice thing is to know that God is listening in and He's okay with our feelings: fear, grief, indescribable sadness, confusion, loss of control— all those things you might expect. Then God takes all that and replaces it with peace for the moment, trust in Him, and joy in the middle of it all. Who knows how He does it! But it happens.

So, for now, all is okay. Big stuff is on the way and we're taking it a day at a time. If you talk to us later this week, we'll be pretty tightly wound, I'm sure. Probably the best thing you can do for us is to pray for us to have peace each day. Thanks for walking with us through all this. You are His hands and feet, and hugging arms.

We love you,

Annette and James

P.S. James has been watching me type this, and just said, "Annette, I'm scared." I quickly looked his way, wondering what he meant. With an odd look in his eyes while gazing at my very bald and uncovered head, he simply said, "I'm getting used to the way you look." I'm soooooooooooooo glad we can laugh together!!!

Wednesday, 16 August

James is gone to church tonight. I've been so tired all day I decided to stay home. Thought I would take a short nap, but as soon as he closed the door, I started crying. The thought of having a breast cut off is frightening. The thought of general anesthesia is frightening; never have liked it. There's always a small chance that something could go wrong. I would be fine to wake up in heaven, but what it would do to James makes me cry. I remember feeling this same way each time I've faced outpatient surgery, so I guess this is no different in that regard. The circumstances are just more serious. This is not elective, nor private, nor affecting just a small part of my being. THIS IS BIG!!!!! Oh, God, help me run to you with my fear so you can replace it with trust in You and your care for me. Help me understand that you have only my best interest in mind. Lord, you just brought to my mind a Dennis Jernigan song:

*I will trust you in the darkness, I will trust
you in life's harshness.
I will trust you, Lord, to guard over my heart.
I will trust you and keep singing, I will trust you,
dearly clinging.
I will trust you and keep bringing you my heart.
Father, I trust you with my heart.*

Lord, I want to trust you; I DO trust you. Nothing else can take away the fear; only You can. Nothing else can put a healing salve on my sadness; only You can. Nothing

else and no one else can lead me through the deep water
of grief; only You can. AND YOU WILL.

As surgery loomed closer, I became more and more nervous about it. My list of things to finish at home and at work in preparation of being out of commission for a few weeks was still somewhat undone. Time had run out and there was nothing left but waiting – and waiting makes me nervous. Sunday morning before surgery dawned on another hot Oklahoma day and my nerves were tightly wound. I felt like a long-tailed cat in a room full of rocking chairs!

Sunday, 20 August

 It's 9:30 p.m. before surgery tomorrow. I have run the gamut of emotions during the last 48 hours: nervous, dread, calm, fear, more dread, increased nervousness. But, praise the Lord, during church tonight I was given a huge sense of peace. It was about 6:30 and we were having prayer time, focusing on other needs as well as my own. Pastor Jim invited others to surround me and place their hands on my shoulders or head during prayer. During the prayer God acted! It was nothing audible; I heard no voice from God. I simply remember taking a deep breath and realizing the heavy weight of fear and dread was gone. I was having a hard time this morning and after-noon; felt little control over my emotions. Although I am a little apprehensive, it's nothing compared to earlier today. I am in God's hands; there's no better place to be.

 I have a few more things to do before going to bed. I should try to clear off the dresser, but it might be more than I can tackle tonight. I am so tired, having not slept much the last two nights. Hopefully, I'll be able to sleep pretty good tonight. Tomorrow's a big day.

Surgery went very well. Everyone at Deaconess Hospital was just wonderful. When I arrived in the surgery area things were a little hectic, as it was their first day in the newly remodeled area. They got me settled in my cubicle and did the usual blood pressure check, change of clothes, and verified that I didn't eat or drink anything that morning. Someone from anesthesia came to talk about the drugs they would use. I made sure he knew that the gas in the nose was fine, but to absolutely *not* put the mask on my face before I was "out" because that freaks me out. So he said they'd use some Versed to relax me first.

When they wheeled me into the surgery suite, all I remember is helping get myself onto the table and a strap going over my shins. That's when I realized how narrow the operating table was! The anesthesiologist took my right arm and placed it on a table extension, telling me he would give me the Versed and would "see me later." That's it; that's all I remember until the recovery room where people were talking all around me, but not to me. I must have made a noise or something because a nurse was looking into my face and saying my name. I'm not sure how long I was there, but I felt cold and was shivering, so they wrapped me in warm blankets. How wonderful! After some time, I remember the gurney started to move and they told me they were taking me to my room ... but I don't remember the journey—only seeing James' face as we went through a doorway. I don't even remember being moved to the bed, but obviously it happened.

When I finally came around, I was asking for food, and received a small bowl of really strong chicken broth. I took one spoonful and promptly threw it up. After that, they had me on a liquid diet — gross!!!! I got jell-o (lemon, orange, lime), very bland soup, custard (which I hate), a cream-of-wheat looking blob for breakfast on Tuesday, more soup, and all the crackers I could ever want. If only I could have smuggled in something solid, but I really didn't even think of it until later.

James stayed with me all day Monday, as did Mama. They took good care of me, since I really didn't move very much until later in the day. Flowers were delivered. People came to visit but I was asleep and never knew they were there.

I remember being relieved that the surgery was over, and being very, very tired. Probably the usual adrenaline letdown after a big event. The incision was completely covered by a very large bandage ... going from middle-chest to the far left side of my back. I had a drain bulb in, which the nurses cared for and later explained what to do with it when I got home. They had me pumped full of medicine, so I really didn't hurt unless I moved my arm too much. And only a little bit was too much.

I went home late in the day on Tuesday, after surgery on Monday morning. By that time I was ready for my own bed, some real food and uninterrupted sleep. The nurses who took care of me were outstanding, but part of their job was to check vital signs regularly. As anyone who has spent at least one night in a hospital knows, it is just not a good place to get some rest.

People brought food to the house. Someone loaned me several books; another brought a bag of movies. There were cards arriving daily. Never have I felt so loved by a group of people! All I had to do was rest and concentrate on recovery. My mom came over each day and stayed until James got home from work. Priceless!!

The follow-up appointments with the surgeon showed that the incision was healing nicely and there were no complications. One disappointing note was that reconstructive surgery would be more difficult. I had elected to defer reconstruction to a later date so that nothing would interfere with future radiation treatments. (An implant does not automatically mean trouble during radiation but I didn't think that I could deal with that at this time, so decided to wait.)

The surgeon had me start a series of at-home exercises to assist my shoulder in returning to full range of motion. Our bodies really are amazing things! I will admit to being a so-so patient on this regard until I heard someone's story about how she couldn't reach to the top shelf in her kitchen. Back to the exercises! Thankfully, I now have only slight pain when I stretch a little too far.

Recovery at home was mostly uneventful. I stayed at home until the third week, when James offered to take me for a ride in the car. I was feeling good enough to be stir-crazy and the thought of getting out sounded wonderful! It only took about four miles for me to regret ever leaving the house and then we had to cover the same four miles to get back home! Even with a pillow to support my arm, the vibrations of the car shook my insides and made everything hurt. It was another week before I tried that again. By then, things were much better and I was looking forward to returning to work.

It was during one of the follow-up appointments with the surgeon that I realized I really didn't like him. While he was technically excellent, I felt he was patronizing me and not answering my questions completely. Since the surgery was behind me, I chose to not press the issue, but I decided that if I ever again needed the services of a surgeon, I would find someone else.

The post-surgery pathology report revealed a Stage III cancer, rather than the Stage II reported on the biopsy done in June. It also showed seven of seven lymph nodes already invaded with cancer cells. My third cycle of chemotherapy was coming up in mid-September and Dr. Hollen was beginning to talk about other types of therapy. One of them was called a Stem Cell Transplant. What I had thought would be a fairly routine treatment schedule changed with this pathology report and I was about to be introduced to the world of high dose chemotherapy.

FIVE

Insurance and Inspiration

Cycle four of Adriamycin and Cytoxan was given on October 11, 2000. Dr. Hollen had sent me home from the third cycle with an armload of information about something called a Stem Cell Transplant (or Reinfusion). Since seven of seven lymph nodes were already invaded with cancer I was at a higher risk for future recurrence. In my meeting with Dr. Hollen prior to cycle four being administered, I told him I wanted to talk with the doctors who were in charge of the transplants. While I had reviewed the brochures, I still had many questions and much apprehension about the procedure.

On October 16, James and I met with Dr. Brian Geister for a consultation. He spent the next hour going over many statistics comparing standard chemotherapy with Stem Cell Transplant following High Dose Chemotherapy. At the time, there were differing views on the efficacy of such a procedure. I was encouraged that he seemed to be giving me both sides of the coin rather than trying to talk me into a major physical and financial event.

We discussed the procedure itself. The most succinct way I can describe it is this: It is a specific and highly toxic plan to take you as close to death as possible and then bring you back. The high dose chemotherapy would literally kill my blood and hopefully any random cancer cells remaining in my body. The subsequent reinfusion of stem cells would be the basis to rebuild my blood count back to a normal range.

Dr. Geister and Dr. Romeo Mandanas are partners in Western Oklahoma Blood and Marrow Transplants. They have put together a small but highly specialized team to oversee outpatient Stem Cell Transplants. Studies have been showing that it is often healthier for a patient to recover from high dose chemotherapy while staying at home as opposed to being hospitalized for a month. Since my home is only six blocks from their treatment center, I could be considered for the procedure as an outpatient.

The major question to answer was, "how much better would my prognosis be by using adjuvant high dose chemotherapy with stem cell rescue?" While I considered my options, I continued with the original chemotherapy plan and had the first cycle of Taxol in early November.

Just a few days after the consultation with Dr. Geister, I attended a weekend retreat for women, sponsored by my church's district. As more than 300 ladies from all over northwest Oklahoma gathered at a hotel in Oklahoma City, I sensed it would be a good event. There was so much cancer-related information rolling around in my head and I longed for a break from thinking about it and my uncertain future. We started with a time for laughter and some praise and worship music, followed by the special speaker, Janine Tartaglia-Metcalfe. She began by reading a scripture portion from the Old Testament Book of Isaiah, chapter 43. It says:

> *"But now, this is what the Lord says – he who created you, O Jacob, he who formed you, O Israel. 'Fear not, for I have redeemed you; I have summoned you by name. You are mine. When you pass through the waters, I will be with you; and when you pass through the rivers, they will not sweep over you. When you walk through the fire, you will not be burned; the flames will not set you ablaze. For I am the Lord, your God, the Holy One of Israel, your Savior ... Do not be afraid, for I am with you.' "*

Wham! God had my undivided attention! There was no audible voice, no shaft of light from the heavens, but the truth of this statement pierced into my heart like nothing I had ever experienced. All I could do was sit and weep while she continued with her message for the evening. I remained focused on what God was saying to me through those first verses even as she used other scripture portions and presented a very inspirational message about getting through life's storms. God confirmed to me that things would be okay. I didn't receive a promise of healing or avoiding further treatment, but I did receive – without a doubt – the absolute assurance that because God had called me *by name*, He was going to be with me through it all.

When the evening session concluded, I found Janine to ask her a question. You see, this women's retreat had originally been scheduled for January and I wanted to know if this was the same message she had planned for that time. She told me that it was not the same ... that sometime in the summer she had begun planning for this "new" time and sensed that God would be pleased for her to use a different opening message than the one she had planned for January. Wow! This was another confirmation that God was/is in the "business" of customizing encouragement for his beloved people!

The next week I called my doctors and told them I wanted to do the Stem Cell Transplant. It was easy to talk about; much harder to do. There were many tests and procedures that had to be done, insurance to be pre-certified, and more planning to be off work for another month.

6-8 November

Tests and more tests: brain scan (yes, I have one), bone scan, chest x-ray, lung function test, bone marrow biopsy, collect urine for a day to test my kidneys (that was interesting), heart pumping test. All of this to see if I'm healthy enough to endure high dose chemotherapy and the Stem Cell Transplant.

14 November

Good news!! All the tests from last week came back negative for cancer anywhere else. Praise the Lord! Now I'm just waiting to see what the insurance company says.

Even though I had been so overwhelmed with God's love for me at the women's retreat and felt comfortable with the plan for high dose chemotherapy, part of me was still scared. I mean, no one really *wants* to put themselves in a position where they might die from what is supposed to save them!

It seemed like every time I would succumb to the anxiety of preparation, God would bring something to encourage my spirit. One of these things was a song made popular by Kathy Troccoli, "My Life Is In Your Hands." Even the title is a statement of faith! Everywhere I turned, I heard this song and was reassured by it. When my pastor asked me to share my testimony at our church's annual Thanksgiving dinner, I agreed, but only if I could sing the testimony. Here are the lyrics to the song that has so much meaning for me:

Life can be so good, life can be so hard,
Never knowing what each day will bring to where you are.
Sometimes I forget, sometimes I can't see
That whatever comes my way, you'll be with me.
My life is in your hands. My heart is in your keeping.
I'm never without hope, not when my future is with you.
My life is in your hands and though I may not see clearly
I will lift my voice and sing 'cause your love does amazing things.
Lord, I know my life is in your hands.
Nothing is for sure, nothing is for keeps,
All I know is that your love will live eternally.
So I will find my rest and I will find my peace
Knowing that you'll meet my every need.

When I'm at my weakest oh, you carry me.
Then I become my strongest, Lord, in your hands.
My life is in your hands and though
I may not see clearly
I will lift my voice and sing 'cause your love
does amazing things.
Lord, I know my life is in your hands.
I trust you Lord, my life is in your hands.

This song became my affirmation of faith that I needed. Whether waking in the middle of the night or while waiting for yet another procedure this was the reminder I needed that, no matter what, I was in good hands.

Tuesday, 21 November

I am so angry! Today I got word from the insurance company that they will pay for a stem cell transplant, but only if I go to an NCI-sponsored clinical trial – and there are none in OKC. They are in San Antonio, Houston, and Tulsa. I am frustrated that the insurance company would send me to a place for treatments, only to tell me they won't pay for the same place to offer additional treatment. Now I have to decide if I'm ready to fight their decision. Tonight, I'm not. I'm totally drained and have no fight in me. Maybe it will be better tomorrow.

I spent a couple of hours a few nights ago searching the internet for info on Stem Cell Transplant and what different sources say about it. Some say it helps prevent breast cancer recurrence; some are not so sure. So what's the big deal about which group sponsors the clinical trial? My insurance company has a "policy" that they will only authorize places sponsored by National Cancer Institute. Why? What right do they have to say I have to travel away from home and go to people whom I do not know? Why will they not authorize doctors I already know? What is different about the clinical trials they are doing? Different drugs? WHAT IS THE DEAL HERE!

A letter that explains all this is supposed to be arriving any day. I will read it and see what, if any, options it gives. Alisa at CCA said one course of action might be to consult with the OK State Insurance Commissioner. Apparently, they have dealt with this before and are knowledgeable about how to proceed. But, again, that means a fight and I don't know if I'm up to it. She said she really didn't want me to have the bad news, but felt like postponing the call wouldn't be right.

*I called the insurance company, but the lady couldn't tell me "why" to any of my questions. I'm sure I sounded rude to her, even as I was trying to keep a rein on my emotions, while at the same time wanting her to know that emotions are involved. She wants me to call these three cities and find out what they offer regarding accommodations, etc. I finally got her to understand that leaving OKC is **not** an option. I have such a strong support system here that has helped me in extraordinary ways. How could I possibly consider taking only one person—and it couldn't be James—to a strange city and staying there for most of a month? When she said I sounded angry, I told her of course I was angry ... that she had effectively made my decision for me to not have the transplant done. When* *the conversation was finished, there were no answers and I felt no better about anything.*

29 November

I had my second cycle of Taxol today. I talked to Dr. Hollen about upcoming procedures and more treatments so he wasn't surprised when I told him I've been somewhat depressed. He said they've been giving me enough medicines to mess with my brain, so it's no wonder I don't feel right. I may opt to take an anti-depressant but didn't want to start that today.

I'm still waiting to hear from the insurance company.

13 December — e-mail to friends

Ready for another epic from Annette?

It's an icy Wednesday evening ... no church tonight! While I'm waiting for the presidential candidates to speak, I want to write about the wonderful things God has been doing in the last couple of weeks concerning my cancer treatments.

I think I mentioned before that the only thing holding me back from the Stem Cell Transplant was word that it would be covered by insurance. It could be a long story, but suffice it to say that after first denying my treatment here in Oklahoma City, they were willing to work out a case rate. Case rate means that they cover all the charges, up to a certain amount. I don't pay anything. Amazing, isn't it? I don't understand the world of health insurance and how their decisions are made. All I know is that they wanted me to travel to Houston or San

Antonio or Tulsa for a transplant in another facility. I simply refused to do that and told them so, rather firmly, I might say. It was just a few days later that I was informed the case rate had been negotiated. {I am coming to believe that God works in and through a strong will that is submitted to HIS will. In different circumstances and ways, this has happened to me before. Some might call it being bossy or assertive, but I think it's more of being willing to ask lots of questions, clearly state a preferred outcome, and then leave the results in God's hands.}

Anyway, once that was settled, James and I met with yet another doctor on the transplant team. He's the head of the whole thing. He didn't say anything we had not heard before, but we walked out of that meeting with a time line for December and January.

First off, I have been given shots of a drug called Neupogen to promote the rapid growth of white blood cells. I had shots all last week. They used little tiny needles, so the shots didn't hurt, but I had to go in every day. Even with valet parking, that takes most of an hour. If you've ever had the flu, you know what I felt like all last week— lots and lots of intense body aches, a little fever, and not much sleep. (Science lesson: The body aches during illness because it's generating a lot more white blood cells to fight the illness. All that happens inside the bones.) One of the worst side effects of the shots was insomnia. I didn't sleep more than about 4-5 hours any night last week. The weird thing was that I wasn't sleepy during the day, just very tired.

This week, I was scheduled for leukapheresis—a fancy word that means they would extract stem cells (immature cells) from my blood, returning the rest of it back to me. Normal procedure is expected to be four hours a day for anywhere from 2-4 days. I showed up at Oklahoma Blood Institute Monday morning, ready to go. They hooked me up to the machine and there I sat for four hours. It didn't hurt, but my face and hands went numb from calcium loss, just like they warned me. That was a strange sensation but all the feeling came back by late afternoon. I had been telling the doctors, nurses, and anyone else who would listen that I was shooting to get it done in one session. (Like I could do something to make it happen!) They said that is highly unusual, but it had been done before.

I did it! While there on Monday, they checked my white blood count level. Normal, healthy people have a white count of about 10,000 ... mine was 97,200 ... almost 10 times as high as usual. Everyone was quite surprised and said something about "a new record high." The usual procedure is for the patient to return the next morning, prepared to stay for another go-round, so there I was again Tuesday morning. No need to stay! In their measurement units for the stem cell transplant, they needed "five" for my body mass ... they got nine! According to OBI, only one person in 100 finishes leukapheresis in just one treatment. So, yes, I do feel pretty special!

Can you believe it? I was so excited that God had blessed me with this wonderful gift!!! I actually jumped for joy there in the waiting room and my hat nearly came off. My remarks the previous few days had been more than simply positive thinking, though I can't say I actually had a strong sense of faith that God would bless me in this specific way. What I had been seeking, though, was a confirmation in my spirit that I was headed down the right path of treatment. (The doctors had told me that there were "jumping off" points along the way, if I felt like changing my mind.) Wow! What a way to confirm that God is working in my body through the use of medicine! So the shots promoted the blood cells to grow. That's good. I just want to witness to the truth that it is God who created it all in the first place.

No more shots or procedures until January 3rd. That's when I have 3 days of high dose chemotherapy, followed by the reinfusion of my stem cells on January 8. Then I rest at home (no visitors) for most of January while my blood rebuilds and energy returns.

So many are continuing to pray for me and I am thankful. Now you can celebrate with me a specific and wonderful blessing! How would I ever make it through all this without my wonderful extended family? I don't think it would be possible. I love you!

SIX

Stem Cell Transplant
(Reinfusion)

I would begin high dose chemotherapy on January 3, 2001. At first Dr. Mandanas didn't understand why I did not want to start treatment in mid-December, as all the tests were finished and the central line catheter was in. His staff enjoyed teasing him that while it might be acceptable in the Philippines (his home country) to miss Christmas with one's family, here in Oklahoma we tend to see things a different way! He was very gracious about my decision to wait and didn't force the issue at all. That was the first time I saw that underneath the very intelligent and professional exterior, he really is quite a pushover ... at least on patient's decisions that aren't life threatening.

James and I tried to complete a redecorating job of one of our bedrooms so it could be my "recovery room." About halfway through December, we realized it was much more work than we anticipated, so we literally closed the door on it and made other plans. We knew that I would have to sleep behind closed doors to keep our cat away from me at night. She had developed the annoying habit of pouncing on my uncovered hands and would sometimes bite me. Obviously, that would be absolutely prohibited with a compromised immune system. Since cats don't usually change their behavior, we made sure we had a plan!

We purchased a trundle bed and placed it in the living room for the month of January. James would sleep there at night and I could rest on it when I came home from treatments. At bedtime I would retire to our bedroom and close the door. We even worked out a call system in case I needed help – I would knock on the wall at the head of our bed and James would come running. We were ready!

Since my immune system would be compromised there were some things I could not eat – no fresh fruit or veggies, only things that were fully cooked. Even fresh flowers were banned from the house. Oddly enough, I could still pet my cat, as long as I was *very* careful that she didn't scratch or bite me.

Sunday, 7 January

I started the high dose chemo last Wednesday. The first day was not bad; just felt like it was more of the same ... at least it seemed that way at first. I arrived there about 8:45 and was greeted by Pam Barnes and Barbara Underwood, who would be our two nurses most of the day. There are also two other stem cell patients going through this. We were all a little nervous, but quickly set at ease.

James was with me for a while (he's still not working steadily because of the snow and ice), then he left and Mama came up with some lunch and stayed through the afternoon. I got home about 3:30 and laid down on the bed in the living room, where I slept. The anti-nausea meds make me sleepy. They use a combination of Benadryl, Ativan, and Dexodran ... thus the name "BAD pump." It's in a little suitcase with wheels and I stayed hooked up to one catheter lumen overnight. The other lumen was a saline solution, set to give me three liters of liquid over 14 hours' time. They know that dehydration is a real threat, so no time is wasted in offsetting it.

Wednesday's highlight was, of course, the Orange Bowl National Championship game with Oklahoma University and Florida State University. I really wasn't sure OU had the stuff to win in Florida, but it was no contest. The OU defense absolutely dominated the FSU offense. Final score: OU 13, FSU 2. That's a great way to start the new year!!

Thursday was more of the same. Nona-Sue Mellish took me to the clinic and stayed all day. It was mostly uneventful. I napped a little, talked some, but am beginning to feel really tired. The high dose effects are kicking in.

Thursday night I started throwing up and was having trouble eating. I could swallow okay; it's just that nothing seemed to set well in my stomach. I hit my "dose" button for some extra relief, but it was a rough night. Friday at lunch, Mama brought me a turkey sandwich from the hospital cafeteria. I took one bite and threw up. So, it was back to crackers and juice. They gave me some I.V. meds

*(phenergan was one), which really put me to sleep. I
barely remember getting home. Friday evening, there was
more vomiting.*

*Yesterday (Saturday) when I went to the weekend
clinic location, I was pretty wiped out. Dr. Mandanas was
there and he changed the dosage on my pump and gave
me a different kind of I.V. medicine. That sure helped. No
more vomiting and I've been able to eat a little bit of real
food. I just hope I'm not driving James nuts with the need
for help. Today, though, I feel like I can do a few things
for myself, but I must be careful not to push it too far.*

Monday, 8 January

*Stem Cell Reinfusion Day!!!!! Mama and I were at the
clinic by 8:45 and the proceedings began. They gave me
some pre-meds (Benadryl, Lorazepam, Dexamethasone,
and Anzemet) to offset nausea and any allergic reaction
to the DMSO that the stem cells are stored in. Since my
cells were harvested in one session, they had been
divided into four bags to be returned to me. I had to ver-
ify that it was my name on the bags and sign a paper
before they got things started. It was like any other I.V.
drip until an awful taste settled in my mouth and I felt so
sick! I started heaving but passed out almost immediately and do not remember most of the morning. I can't
describe the taste of the DMSO. All I know is that it felt
like something was foaming from my mouth. When I
came to, the nurses assured me that it's all very normal.
Who cares? It was so gross. It's been suggested that it
was like a strong garlic taste or maybe creamed corn,*

STEM CELL TRANSPLANT (REINFUSION) | 67

but I wouldn't put either of those names on the taste. Garlic breath is better than that!

Today I also began injections of Leukine, which is made to stimulate growth of very young cells in my bone marrow. If I react to it like I did the Neupogen, my blood counts should take off in good order. That would be nice. By mid-afternoon, all that was done and Mama brought me home. Evening was mostly uneventful, although I felt like I'd been beaten up and thrown away.

Tuesday, 9 January
Mama and I were talking today while at the clinic. This would have been her parents' 89th wedding anniversary. They married in 1922, having waited until Anna Baldwin was 19 years old. Her beau, Arthur Brandon, wanted to make sure that Rev. and Mrs. Baldwin wouldn't prohibit the marriage. I've enjoyed talking to Mama these hours we've had together. We talk about family or Jesus or even stuff that won't matter tomorrow. I am so blessed to have her here. Thank you, Lord, for giving me such a precious gift!

This was not such a bad day. Nothing unusual went on. No vomiting in about 24 hours, so they unhooked me from both the BAD pump and fluid pump. I'm free! I can walk somewhere without my tag-along getting in the way! Considering that the alternative was to be hospitalized a few days, I really didn't mind the pumps. They were definitely good things to have.

I stink. The DMSO is dissipating from my body and I smell awful! James says he can smell it the minute he

walks in the house. Nurse Barbara says it will go away in
a couple of days.

Wednesday, 10 January
Ugh. I feel awful. I'm nauseated. I've got diarrhea. My
insides have turned to water and Imodium is not helping.
I think the high dose side effects are in full swing now. My
blood counts today showed that the high dose chemo is
certainly at work to kill off anything that reproduces
quickly, including cancer.
White blood cells: 0.5 (Normal is 4.8-10.8 for women—
that's to say 4800 to 10800; I've been on the higher end.)
Platelets: 76 (Normal is 130-400; read that 13000-
40000.)
They're not so concerned about red blood cells, as
they do not dramatically drop like the other two.
James went to church, after making sure I felt okay. I
thought an hour or so alone might be a good thing. Well,
I was wrong. He hadn't been gone very long when I just
started bawling. I couldn't stop crying for quite a while. I
have no idea why I cried, or if there even was a reason.
But after a while, the tears stopped and I felt better. By
the time he got home, I was emotionally even. Maybe this
is why the doctors have me on Prozac, to help eliminate
frequent dramatic swings of emotion.

Thursday, 11 January
Ohhhhhhhhhh. My counts have plummeted and I feel
so bad. This is where my trust in God has got to kick in,
'cause I have no energy to fight. I know others are praying

for me and that's my source of hope. Nona-Sue was with me again today. I think I kept her hopping with requests for juice or crackers or something to nibble on, or the need to go find a nurse. Nurse Barbara kept reassuring me that this was supposed to be a puny day, so I was "normal".

White cells: 0.1   Platelets: 59

Friday, 12 January

I thought yesterday was bad. It's been 10 days since high dose chemo started and I'm feeling every bit of it today. James left for work at 7:00 this morning and I was feeling weak, but okay and moving slowly. Mama would arrive about 8:00, so I was getting ready to bathe when gut cramps suggested a different priority. So there I was sitting on the toilet, dealing with diarrhea as usual, when I had a horrible bout of cold chills. There was cold sweat running down my face and neck, arms and legs. I was shivering uncontrollably. I was crying and so scared I'd pass out and hurt myself. I wanted to sit on the floor, but the diarrhea continued, so I just held on to the toilet paper holder.

As best I can figure this went on for about 20 minutes, then the doorbell rang. I made a very slow walk to the door. Thankfully, there were no accidents on the way. It was Mama and the storm door latch wouldn't come open. She knew at once that I was in trouble, so she helped me to bed where I stayed until 8:30, when I called the doctor. "Do I have to come in today or can you come to me?" Dr. Geister nicely but firmly said there were no options—I had to get there. So we got me dressed and a wheel chair was waiting at the door. I must have really looked bad, because eyes were popping out of heads from the nurses in the treatment room. Both Drs. Geister and Mandanas came to see me after the blood work had been done. My white count today is at 0.0—which would explain the episode in the morning. Platelets are at 35.

Saturday/Sunday, 13–14 January

Since my immune system is so compromised, I am not allowed to leave the house. Home health came out to draw blood work, give me a Leukine shot, and check my vital signs. I actually felt very good on Saturday—even to the point of putting on some make-up. James cooked a frozen pizza for lunch and I had two pieces. My tongue is white from the chemotherapy and I really don't taste much, but I am soooooo tired of mashed potatoes, Jell-o, and other bland foods. For supper, he fetched a Pollo Monterrey dinner from Las Palomas. I could only have the chicken with mushrooms and cheese, and the refried beans, but oh, my—what a treat for my medicated taste buds!! My taste buds don't work very well, so maybe it was all in my mind, but that food was so good!

Dr. Geister made a house call Saturday morning. He seemed surprised that I felt so much better than just 24 hours before. Another home health nurse came back in the evening to give me a transfusion of platelets. So far, though, I've not needed a full blood transfusion. That's good.

Sunday morning, Dr. Geister called from his mobile phone and asked some questions. He was trying to get to church and since I felt so good, it seemed unnecessary for him to come to the house. The home health nurse came by and did the usual, but I did not need any platelets today. Mama was with me this morning. She ended up coming back in the evening, too. After James left for church, my fever went up and I felt a little wobbly. I had promised them both that if I felt unsteady, I'd call. Later in the evening, she said, "It only took 7 minutes to get here. I guess traffic was light." I think Mama has a lead foot!

Monday-Wednesday, 15–17 January
    Fever! Constant, debilitating fever. For a normal healthy person a temperature of 99.6 is not all that high, but mine went up to 100.7 and was unbearable. James called Dr. Geister at 2:10 a.m. Tuesday because it had reached the "magic number" of 100.5. After a series of questions, Doc said it sounded like the Leukine shots are revving up my bone marrow, so a natural side effect is for the body to think it has an infection and try to kill it with a fever. So, the fever in this case is good. I'm trying to grab hold of that concept, but it just feels so bad. I feel like I can't do anything and this is beginning to be a longer, harder ordeal than I can cope with. James is so good, but I'm probably driving him nuts with all my asking for help.
    Every day now I am getting two kinds of I.V. antibiotics: Vancomycin and Levofloxacin. The latter is given first and takes about an hour to drip; the first one takes about two hours. Every day my catheter dressing is changed and I get a shot of Leukine. My temperature, blood pressure and weight are written down.

My blood counts have been:

Mon., Jan. 15:   *White count: 0.1 — up from 0.0 on*
                          Jan. 12!! Progress!
                          Platelets: 21 — still falling, but that's
                          normal
Tues., Jan. 16:   *White count: 0.2—double from*
                          yesterday!!
                          Platelets: 20 ... but still no need for a
                          transfusion (doctors are surprised)
Wed., Jan. 17:   *White count: 0.6—tripled from*
                          yesterday!!
                          Platelets: 36 — up from yesterday

I am amazing the transplant team again with my response to the Leukine shots. Though they target different cells, my body is responding the same as when I was given Neupogen. This has been so hard, the fever is just so persistent and I have no energy to fight, but every day there is encouraging news. I know it's because of the prayers of many people all over the globe.

Mama and I were wondering Tuesday if there would be any possible way to assemble a list of people—by name—who have been praying for me. It's a daunting task that I can't do now, but it would be an incredible, concrete testimony to God's faithfulness.

Wednesday, James was with me all day because it snowed and he couldn't work. Sometime in the afternoon, Daddy called and said Mama had broken her right wrist during a fall inside the house! She's going to be okay, but is very sore all over. Doctor said it's a clean break and will not require surgery. She, of course, feels bad because she can't take care of me now. I talked to her later in the day and she sounded medicated and tired, but okay.

Thursday, 18 January
Tami Waits came by this morning and took me to the clinic. She stayed a while then went to check on her sister-in-law, who is having back surgery today. The morning passed quietly, though a persistent queasy feeling left me uncomfortable. I probably should have said something to the nurse, but didn't. I tried eating two different kinds of crackers, but had to stop after one bite each. About 11:30 Tami returned with my choice of lunch—an Arby's roast beef sandwich. It only took three bites and up it came, along with the Jell-o I had consumed an hour before.

So, they slapped some medicine in my I.V.: phenergan, again. It is an effective drug, but I can't stand what it does to my brain—puts me to sleep.

When my fever went up to 102.9, Nurse Barbara brought me some Tylenol. I'm sure it was very amusing to anyone who would have just walked in on the scene: I'm in bed, holding a cup of pudding in my left hand. I've just been given a pill to swallow, and on its way to my mouth, I go back to sleep. The nurse wakes me and I finally get the pill down; she, of course, holds the cup of water and I sip through a straw. Otherwise, it would have been a disaster. The whole thing is repeated with the second pill. All the while, I'm still holding the cup of pudding.

Sometime later, I awake to find the pudding gone and have no idea who took it away. I threw up again in mid-afternoon, so they gave me even more phenergan and I was knocked out even longer.

*Finally, around 5:30, we were able to leave the clinic. Someone wheeled me downstairs; I have no idea which nurse it was. They helped me into the car and we got home. I remember walking into the house, taking off my coat and falling onto the bed in the living room. That's it. I don't know when James got home or when Tami left the house. I **do** know I am very blessed to have a friend like Tami.*

James did not go to the church board meeting. I needed someone to stay with me and he was not going to let anyone else do it. Late in the evening, he got me to bed. I actually slept better than I had in several nights. So that side effect of the phenergan did help me.

Good news with my blood count—it continues to increase rapidly:

White count: 1.5 — up from 0.6 yesterday

Platelets: 52 — up from 36 yesterday

Friday, 19 January

This has been a good day. Very little nausea and I'm eating a little better. They have gone back to Neupogen, hoping to get away from the fevers. It's not as likely to produce fever, although bone pain is probable. It was a short visit to the clinic. No antibiotics are needed, because my counts are up high enough:

White count: 3.5 — again, double from the day before

Platelets: 64

Tami and I were leaving the clinic by about 10:00—wow! She took me home, and left me by myself only when I promised that I really felt okay. Not weak and faintish or nauseated. She ran some errands, then brought back some lunch: a Wendy's hamburger with lettuce and tomato! My food restrictions have been lifted, so I can have fresh fruit and veggies again. I ate about half the burger, along with a Coke. After a couple of hours, she decided I really wasn't going to throw up, so she left me alone.

By mid-afternoon, my fever was up slightly and my legs were hurting. It took a while for me to realize what was going on. The Neupogen was kicking in. So I just took two Tylenol and then took a nap.

Saturday, 20 January

I've been alone at home all day. I felt good enough to stay awake and watch the entire presidential inauguration on television. James is working; no visits or calls from doctors or home health nurses. Just the cat and me, keeping each other company. I've had a slight fever, controlled with more Tylenol.

I am beginning to understand what the nurses meant when they said there would be short bursts of energy, but I should pace myself. Today I did the laundry, but after each load was in the washer or dryer, I had to sit down for a while. My muscles hurt and I feel incredibly weak. Not faint, just like a real weenie. James and I had talked about going to Applebee's for an early supper. Even if he had not worked late, I wouldn't have made it. Just the idea of leaving the house was too much for today. I am hoping I feel good enough for church in the morning.

Sunday, 21 January

I went to church! I walked in late so I wouldn't have to talk to anyone. Just getting dressed wore me out ... I felt really shaky by the time I made that long one-block drive down the street. When I walked into the back of the Sanctuary, Bob and Donna Olmstead were near the door and broke into broad smiles when they saw me. I let Bob escort me to the soundboard; I felt that wobbly on my feet. Oh, how wonderful it was to be in the house of the Lord! After the service, James guarded me closely, not letting people get within hugging distance. It probably would have been okay, since my white count is up, but I just didn't want to take the risk. Many came by and greeted me. It was so good to see everyone again. I felt like I've been gone for ages.

Monday, 22 January

Today, there was a change of pace. When I arrived at the clinic—by myself, I might add—there were no medicines scheduled for me. They took some blood and sent it to the lab. My white count was up to 11,400. Good grief, I sure do respond to the Neupogen! Then I got the news—no treatment of any kind today. No antibiotics, no I.V. fluids, no shots— nothing! That's weird. After such intense care for the last 2-1/2 weeks, it was strange to not have them do anything.

After a while, Dr. Mandanas came in to remove my catheter. He had me turn my head to the left. He said it was to relax the neck, but I think it's more for the patient not to see the doctor strain when he pulls. Anyway, he told me it would hurt a little, and pulled hard. Ouch, it hurt, more than a little, but not enough to make me scream ... just groan a little and take a deep breath. He was concerned about hurting me. Sometimes, he said, the skin grows around the catheter, requiring a surgical removal. As he prepared to pull again, I said a quick prayer that it would come out. It did! It really smarted, to say the least, but after a few minutes I was okay. I had reminded him that I wanted to keep the catheter, so he put it in a bag for me. Later a nurse told me how I could clean it up so the skin particles and blood would be removed. It would be pretty gross to look at it in a month and find yucky stuff growing. We paid good money for that thing and it was part of me for two months. It even had a name: Kate, the Catheter. (Remember, I wasn't getting out much, so I found ways to amuse myself!)

I was sent home with the bag, the rest of a bottle of antibiotics, and instructions to come back on Friday. How strange will that be? The thought crossed my mind that they're just throwing me to the dogs. Of course, that's not true, but it kind of seems that way. So, I just went home, called James and took the rest of the day to relax.

Tuesday, 23 January

I took the car to have it washed, but I forgot to put down the antenna, so now it's broken. It still works, but sits at a funny angle. The weird thing is that I thought of it as I was getting out of the car, but took two steps and forgot. Just a short time away from the house and I tired so quickly. I also noticed that noise and traffic and being around lots of people were making me nervous. Home is a nice haven from all that.

Wednesday, 24 January

This is indeed a red-letter day: I was able to take a shower. How glorious! What an amazing thing it is to have water cascading down my back. Ahhhhhhh. The catheter was placed on December 8 and I tried a couple of times to shower, but the dressing got wet. So it has been close to two months since I stood under running water. Thankfully, the soap I got from Deaconess was such a great thing. At least I never went around feeling stinky and grungy.

Friday, 26 January

I have officially been released from the care of the Transplant Team. Today I met with Dr. Geister for my final appointment. He came in, gave me a big hug, and reviewed the results of my lab work, which is well within the normal range. It's lower than on Monday because of not having any more shots. This means the transplant was successful and my new blood cells are reproducing well.

Dr. Geister spent about 20 minutes with me talking about how I feel today and what will be coming up. He even asked if I was having hot flashes. (The answer is yes.) Understanding that my body has been chemically altered is a big step in realizing what is going on internally. He said it will be about 6 months before my energy and stamina levels return to normal, and that walking briskly for 15 minutes a day, 3 days a week will help (increasing that to 30 minute brisk walks 5 days a week). We talked about the psychological effect of not coming for treatment every day. Many patients actually experience "withdrawal" from the daily care of the transplant process. He said that was very normal and I was always welcome to drop in to see them.

I asked him if he recommended radiation therapy. He took a minute to get my post-surgery pathology report and see what it said. Considering the size and location of the tumor, he strongly suggested I move to the next step. I felt I probably would need radiation, so this was no surprise.

Then we spent a few minutes talking about prayer and what a difference that makes in a patient's recovery process. It was encouraging to me to hear him say how he desires for every patient that they nourish the soul as well as the body and mind. Now I know why, from the very first appointment, I felt he could be trusted for my care.

I went back to work on January 29th, though not full time. I still tired easily and had a tendency to over-exert myself. James and I had some frank discussions about that. It seemed that the first couple of things that got my attention early in the day were all I could deal with and that left me with no energy for time with James. I know we will get through this and am thankful he's being honest with me about his feelings.

Withdrawal from treatment, indeed! It was very strange that I did not have to run up to the clinic for treatment or lab work.

I really did miss it—not the treatments, but the people. Just a few days later the thought came to mind that there was "something" I should be doing. Then I realized it had been some time since I'd had any doctor's appointments. That's what was missing from my schedule. Dr. Geister was right; I was going through withdrawal!

Thursday, 21 February

Yesterday was 6 months since my mastectomy. So much has happened! The scar where my breast was removed has healed well. I suppose it is acceptable, except for the fact that there just is no way to make it "pretty." I still don't like the way the skin is under my arm—like I have two armpits. If I ever wanted to wear a sleeveless shirt, this would make me change my mind for sure! Then there is the extra fat or skin that is on my side. I still don't understand where it came from; only that it was not like that before surgery and my right side isn't that way. The surgeon told me that some women have a second surgery, or additional work during reconstructive surgery, to take care of that problem. For now, I can't even think about someone coming at me with a scalpel.

Monday, 26 February

Last Friday, I met with Dr. Hollen again. We talked about how I'm feeling—mostly good, although too tired for my preference. I've been continuing to have hot flashes, too, so he suggested an increase in the dosage for Prozac. No lab work, but have another appointment in a month.

He also recommended that I meet with a radiation oncologist. I knew that was coming, but really don't want to face another round of treatment. I am so incredibly tired of fighting this thing ... of having to think about what's next. It seems almost unbearable at times.

SEVEN

Radiation & Lymphedema

In some ways, radiation therapy was the hardest of all the treatments I had. Perhaps it was because I had gone back to work and was determined to not leave again. Perhaps it was because I was beginning to feel stronger after the Stem Cell Transplant and now it was time to get involved with another treatment. That took a lot of mental and physical energy out of me. Once the preliminary scans and tests were done, it was determined I would need 42 radiation treatments. That meant five days a week for almost two months!

Monday, 5 March

Had a radiation simulation today. Ouch! I can't be still that long without great distress. Here's the deal: You lay down on a cold, hard slab, with the knees elevated a little by a pillow wedge to ease lower back pain. Then you raise your hand over your head; hold on at a funny-feeling angle. That's when they say "don't move." Don't move? I am not a mannequin and can't NOT move. It took about 1-1/2 hours to do all the CT scan they needed. I was able to move a little, but not much, and was very glad when it was done. Now they will use the scanned image of me to figure out what kind of fields they need for radiation.

Last week I met Dr. Chris Bozarth, a radiation oncologist at Integris Baptist Hospital. After I got over the fact that he looked way too young to even have a clue about what he was doing, we spent about an hour together with him doing most of the talking. (I'm only 43, but this doctor really looks young!) He reviewed my post-surgery pathology report with me and explained, in detail, what the purpose of radiation is and what he hoped to accomplish.

I had never thought about it before, but he said that when surgery is done, it cuts off some of the blood supply to where the tumor was; a natural side effect to the cutting that is done on the body. Chemotherapy can only work where blood goes, which is why radiation is a supplemental treatment. It affects all tissue it reaches. They also have to be careful to shield the heart and lungs during treatments. Since there could be cancer cells remaining in the area of the incision and lymph nodes radiation is the best way to treat it.

He promised me that he really isn't a sadist, but that he knows the radiation is working when my skin starts to burn. *Eeewww. I don't like the sound of that. He also told me that once the treatments begin, I can't put any lotion or creams or anything on that part of my body. If I need something, ask and they'll provide acceptable products.*

Looks like I could begin later this week, but he will let me know after they have determined all the angles and everything they need.

Saturday, 17 March

It was seven years ago today that my mother-in-law passed away. I remember so clearly how those two days were—waiting so long during her surgery, then waiting more after it was over. Maybe it's because I am in the middle of medical attention that the emotions we felt during that time are not too far away right now. Hard to believe it's been that long.

I began radiation treatment last Tuesday. So far, so good. My appointment is scheduled at 4:45 each day, which helps in several ways: I only leave work once and it's easier to find a parking place because so many are leaving the hospital about that time. Plus, I like being able to go home after treatment. They have made so many marks on my chest with a Sharpie that I feel you could play connect-the-dots. Seems like each day it's a different color: red, green, purple, black. Amy, one of the radiation techs, said that after this week, she'll put some little tattoos on me—sort of like freckles—so they won't have to make so many marks every day. The biggest thing that bothers me about it right now is that the marks rub off on my clothes! Hope it comes out in the wash.

Yesterday I saw Dr. Hollen again for a monthly check up. He was pleased with my blood count, so that's good. I have been feeling sick for a few days and he wasn't happy that I had not already called for an earlier appointment. Seems there is a nasty virus going around and I have it. He prescribed some antibiotics to help me fight the stuff, some cough syrup, and 3 days of bed rest. "I don't want to hear about any sightings of 'Typhoid Annette' this weekend." Yes, sir, you don't have to tell me twice. I am getting some rest this weekend, but don't actually feel much better yet.

Thursday, 5 April

Well, it's been awhile since I've written anything. Most days have been the same routine: Get to work around 9:00 and leave at 4:15 for radiation. Each treatment has continued as before, only now my skin is burned and it's pretty uncomfortable to wear clothes. That's not a problem, of course, unless I want to go to work or out in public somewhere.

Dr. Bozarth's nurse, Royce, has given me some cream that helps soothe my skin a little. They also recommend a cortisone cream to ease the itching. At night I can take Benadryl, but not during the day! The entire left side of my chest is red, from the sternum to slightly behind and including the armpit; from my shoulder to just above the waist. I am only half done with radiation. What will I feel like in another 3 weeks?

One of the things I am dealing with now is a return of some emotions. I guess the high dose chemo did a number on my brain, because I don't remember feeling very much until a couple of weeks ago. Maybe it's a part of this whole process with cancer, but sometimes my mind wants to leap to the worst possible scenario, dwelling there for a few minutes on thoughts of being too sick to work and going deep into debt, of dying. Three nights in a row I dreamed some kind of "abandonment" dream—different people had just left me somewhere and I had no way to get back to a safe place like home. Spooky. I'm glad it didn't last longer than 3 nights. I told James about it and we talked a little about that kind of feeling.

I also feel weepy pretty often. It has occurred to me that, while going through chemotherapy, I simply didn't know that emotions had faded. Now that they are returning it is unusual to feel things—anger, sadness, fear. Interesting that I've just written down "negative" emotions. I know God has given me a happy heart even in the middle of all this junk. Maybe He has put other things on hold until I can deal with them better.

This e-mail was sent to friends and family members to keep them updated on my progress:

It's time for another epistle from Annette. I hope this finds all of you rested from your weekend—ha! Why is it we try to pack too much into a few hours on Saturday or Sunday? Maybe some day we'll learn.

It has been a couple of months since I have updated my medical status, so I thought I would do that and also ask for your continued prayers. Late January and most of February was quite wonderful—no needles, no medicine, no procedures. After seven months of chemotherapy and surgery, that was a very nice respite. As the transplant team had forewarned me, I did have a little feeling of being tossed out to fend for myself; but, only for a while.

Late February I started meeting with a Radiation Oncologist, to set out the plan for the next part of my treatment. Again, God answered prayer for a doctor with whom I was comfortable and whose judgment I could trust. Studies show that the usual place for a breast cancer to recur is in the skin nearest the original tumor. My tumor was just underneath the skin, so this would be especially true in my case. The radiation is yet another step in lowering the probability of recurrence. So, plans were made, CT scans were done and I began radiation in mid-March. I go to the radiation department at Baptist each weekday afternoon where I receive both electron and photon radiation. The procedure itself is not painful, except for my arm which sets in a cradle for the treatment time, about 15 minutes. Do you know how h-a-r-d it is to keep an arm still for that long!? It's a real stretch for me to do that, but so far, I'm okay.

What is painful is the accumulating affect of the radiation. Dr. Bozarth said that by the end of the treatments, I'll have a "bad" first degree burn on my skin — and I'm only halfway finished. I have had a bad sunburn only 2 or 3 times in my life, and I must say that I didn't like it—I was very uncomfortable for several days. I have already begun using the special cream given to me and I take Benadryl at night to ease the itchy skin. The doctor and assistants have all reminded me almost daily to use the cream, but not to use any other home-made remedies. They have said, "This part of your skin is ours to treat and care for. Don't do anything to it without our permission." Since I'm trying to be a good patient and not work against the treatment, I'll behave.

Radiation also affects my energy level, which has been moderate at best. So, if you call the office in the morning and the answering machine picks up, you'll know I'm not out playing "hooky" ... although last Monday afternoon it was so nice, I sure wanted to!

Your continued prayers will be needed in the next few weeks. I am so blessed to have a large group of people who are praying for me! There is no way I can express how much this means to me ... your caring hearts are very special. Spread the news as you talk to others who don't have e-mail.

Psalm 94:19: "When anxiety was great within me, your consolation brought joy to my soul."

You are deeply loved,
Annette

As Dr. Bozarth said, radiation got worse—or rather, the effects on my skin got worse. By the fourth week, the burn was more than a little uncomfortable. I realized on Monday, April 9, while at work that I was really hurting a lot, so I asked them about it when I arrived for treatment. Dr. Bozarth winced when he saw the burn, and told me it was a first degree burn and we still had another three weeks to go. (He had changed the treatments to a total of seven weeks; up from six.) Nurse Royce applied some celluloid bandage that would keep the skin from being rubbed raw by clothing or skin-on-skin contact. It's like a stick-on bandage that kept the moisture on the wound. She described it like amniotic fluid is to a baby in the womb—a safe, sterile environment for the new skin to grow. It could not get wet, so I had to return to sponge baths. No showers for a while. She also told me it would begin to stink when it started filling up with stuff; and that when it was ready to come off, it would practically fall off with a gentle tug.

She was right. It stunk really badly!! About two days later I thought everybody around me could smell it, but no one said anything. When I asked Royce about it, she assured me that it really isn't a strong smell ... just a direct line from my armpit to my nose, so it seems really strong to me. She showed me how to remove it and sent me home with a sheet of the bandage, in case it was needed over the weekend.

My treatments continued throughout April. It finally became very routine to check in, change into a gown, and traipse down the hall to the treatment room. Without even realizing it, I reached the point where it all took about 15 minutes. When everything began, Dr. Bozarth had told me my actual appointments would be short, but there was so much measuring and x-raying and adjusting that it took a long time to get to that point.

Funny, on reflection, though I saw the staff every day, it was kind of like a usual doctor's appointment—the staff was very kind, knowledgeable, and thorough in their work ... but not much of a relationship was formed. Quite the opposite of what happens with chemotherapy.

My last day of radiation therapy was Thursday, April 26. When I finished the final treatment, they brought me a purple balloon connected to a yellow "stress ball" character with a smiley face. They also gave me a certificate, stating I had success-fully completed the treatments. It was all very nice, if low key. When I got home, I called Mama and Daddy and yelled into the phone, "I'm finished!" James and I met Jon and Tami for supper at Western Sizzlin' on Meridian for a celebratory dinner. After a few days of recovery from the burn I was finally able to return to work.

Somewhere in the later weeks of radiation, I began to have substantial swelling in my left arm—Secondary Lymphedema. Lymphedema is a condition caused by a malfunction in the lymphatic system. The lymphatic system is made up of the tissues and organs that produce, store, and carry white blood cells that fight infection and other diseases. It includes the bone marrow, spleen, thymus and lymph glands and a network of thin tubes that carry lymph and white blood cells into all the tissues of the body. Lymph fluid removes bacteria and certain proteins from the tissues, along with other functions.

For me, Lymphedema manifests itself by swelling in my left shoulder, arm and hand. I had seven lymph nodes removed dur-ing surgery and what remained of those thin tubes was so badly damaged by radiation therapy that the system literally "backs up" in my left arm.

Arrangements were made for me to have some physical ther-apy to help reduce the swelling. I saw a physical therapist for a few visits, with mixed results from the arm massages. At first it seemed to help but after a couple of weeks, my hand and arm puffed up and did not go back to their normal size. By the mid-dle of June 2001 I was seeing a Lymphedema therapist.

I saw some improvement in the Lymphedema, but there was, and continues to be, a lot involved in daily treatment. I must wear a compression glove and sleeve during the day. It can be uncomfortable and certainly has slowed my typing speed. The relief I feel each evening when the compression garments are removed is significant, if short-lived. Generally, my left arm and hand are "free" for about only 2-3 hours a day.

At night, I wear about 90 feet of bandages on my arm ... and then try to get a good night's sleep! The finger bandages are first. There are two strands of gauze, about an inch wide, which are wrapped around and in between each finger and the thumb in a specified pattern. The gauze crosses over the back of the hand and ends up at the wrist.

Next, a long cotton "stocking" goes over my hand and arm. It has a cut-out for my thumb so I retain fairly good mobility with my hand. Over the stocking is a roll of thin foam which is layered all the way from the hand to the armpit. After that, there are three different widths of Ace-like bandages that are rolled around the hand (between thumb and forefinger) and all the way up the arm. The bandages are held in place with cloth tape. I also use a variety of foam pieces to keep the tissue from becoming hard and fibrous. The entire wrapping process takes my husband about six minutes to complete. I can do it myself, but it takes me about 20 minutes and lots of tape!

The bandages are heavy and restrict movement at the wrist, elbow, and shoulder. Because of this, I often have much pain in the left shoulder and neck area. If you have ever had your arm in a cast, you can understand how uncomfortable it is to have limited movement of your arm. However, unlike a cast that is removed after a few weeks, my arm must be wrapped every night.

People ask me if Lymphedema hurts. Sometimes my arm does ache. Most of the ache, though, is in the shoulder and neck from restricted movement. Having my arm above my head for even a few minutes restricts the nerves and makes my arm and hand tingle.

How long will I have to wear compression garments? I think it will be until God heals me from this disease. I have had several series of intense sessions, from 3 to 6 weeks of almost daily therapy with Lymphedema therapists, and they have produced some good results that did not last very long. As soon as I resumed my regular daily routine, the swelling returned.

Is there a cure for Lymphedema? No. You manage the disease and live your life anyway.

Natural curiosity from others almost never causes me any embarrassment or negative feelings. The struggle comes from the never-ending reality of having one arm significantly larger than the other. Shopping for clothes is a nightmare, as my left arm is often two sizes larger than the rest of me. When I find something that fits correctly, alterations must be made to accommodate the swelling in my left arm. If the fabric isn't stretchy, I will often have to cut the seams so the sleeve is open underneath.

I discovered that I always prefer to put my right shoulder toward the camera for any photo ... just one of my tricks in managing the disease. Most people do not notice the swelling, but when I see a photo with my left arm exposed, it magnifies my own level of discomfort.

You would be amazed at how much you can do with only one hand. I feel like I have mastered the art of cooking and washing dishes with my right hand, with minor balancing help from my left hand. My left hand and arm are fully functional, but I have to be extra careful with the garments. They are expensive and some are not covered by insurance so I try to make them last as long as possible. The compression sleeve and glove must be washed by hand every night and hung up to dry. After all, I wash my hands every day, and those garments go everywhere my hands go!

It's all about routine. I once told a friend that living with Lymphedema is similar to the way my dad manages diabetes. There is no known cure, no surgery to make it go away, so I had to make a choice. I could whine and complain and refuse to take care of my arm or I could make every effort to manage the disease. It does take a lot of time and effort, but it has built itself into my daily life. It's my new normal.

I see a Lymphedema therapist who keeps me informed on the latest in Manual Lymph Drainage massage, orders bandages and compression garments, and keeps me updated on the latest medical news. She is another member of the team of professionals who are helping me through this journey after cancer.

Even with careful management of the disease, I have had several bouts of Cellulitis, an infection of the skin, spending a few days in the hospital three of those times. It presented itself without warning, usually in the middle of the night. When the fever is high and the pain is severe, there's no thought of waiting until the next business day to call my family doctor. Thankfully, we live just blocks away from two very good hospitals.

Once the diagnosis was made in the Emergency Room, antibiotics were administered for about 48 hours through an I.V. and then switched to pill form. During the hospital stays, I was unable to have any compression on my arm as the infected skin was very red (like a bad sunburn) and hot to the touch. It would have made it even worse to cover the arm with all the compression bandages! Cold compresses and keeping the arm elevated with lots of pillows helped to ease the discomfort until the antibiotics kicked in and the swelling was reduced. I am thankful that my family doctor is teaching me how to care for Cellulitis at home. We have an agreement that if it stays within specific parameters, I don't have to rush to the hospital—but I still have to call him first thing the next morning!

I will confess that sometimes it is hard not to have a "pity party" while living with Lymphedema. I just want it to go away. Many have joined my husband and me to pray for my healing. It seems that, for now, God is saying "not yet" to healing but I am looking forward to the day when He says "yes, now is the time!" In the meantime, I must recommit myself to the care and management of the disease and trust the outcome to the One who knows me best. Psalm 91:1-2 says it well:

"He who dwells in the shelter of the Most High will rest in the shadow of the Almighty. I will say of the Lord, 'He is my refuge and my fortress, my God in whom I trust.'"

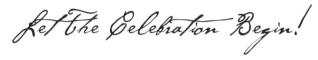

EIGHT

Let The Celebration Begin!

As I looked back over my journal from time to time, I felt that I had written a pretty good narrative about the events that happened from diagnosis through all the treatments. What was much harder was to put my feelings on paper. I guess I'm no different than anyone else facing cancer: I was alternately content with the progress, angry and resentful that I even had to deal with it at all, and sometimes, very scared about the future.

One day I was looking at pictures from the transplant weeks and it was hard to remember it. I wish we had taken more pictures of the whole process. There I was in my little room with the doctor checking my heart and breathing ... but what was I *feeling?* I'm not sure, except for the immediate "pain and suffering" of the day. Maybe that's what selective memory is about ... helping you deal with stuff when you're strong enough to handle it.

I believe with all my heart that God carried me through all this, so I want to choose to be content with the process of emotional health, too. Mom and Dad have said I've always had a happy demeanor, even since infancy. If that is my natural state, I sure don't want to manufacture dark days just because it seems like this has been too easy. Well, not exactly easy, but I've not been completely undone by it all. Sure, there have been many days that I did not want to do anything except stay in bed and try to escape it all. But the stronger desire to return to "normal" won out and I got up and went to work or to do things with James.

On June 15, 2001, James and I hosted a party to thank everyone who helped us get through the worst year of our lives. We mailed invitations to all the medical people and friends who did specific things ... like mow the yard, bring in meals, volunteer for me in the office, drive James to places when he couldn't drive himself, and more. We both took a vacation day to prepare for the party. It was a lot of work but well worth it!

We had been planning the party for months. We wanted to do something special for those who cared for us so well in such a difficult time. But, how in the world could we do that? We finally decided that the only thing we could do was to offer a dinner in their honor and publicly recognize that we would never have made it without them. So, we sent the invitations, ordered a cake and decorated the church fellowship hall with balloons in bright colors. A friend agreed to grill the burgers for us, even bringing his own sauce that made them extra-good. Another friend surprised me with a huge bouquet of absolutely exquisite and richly aromatic red roses from his garden. Others brought some cards with thoughtful words inside. Humorous or sentimental, we treasured them all! I had made some guest registration sheets so we would be able to remember who was there. Almost everyone wrote some kind of note. We had fun reading them later and have kept them.

Shortly after the first anniversary of my diagnosis, I began to ponder the word "remission" and its various meanings. I remember thinking early in my cancer treatment process that the goal would be remission. All the experts say that there is no cure for cancer. The only way to measure a so-called "cure" is to take it one day at a time, fight it with all your might using the full arsenal of treatments, and then let nature take its course.

So that's what I've done—fought it with all I have, both from within and without, and now I have reached the goal: remission. But what does that mean?

The medical definition of remission is: "An abatement or subsiding of the symptoms of a disease."

To be honest this definition really doesn't offer much long-term hope for cancer not recurring. However, my hope is not found in what other people say ... even as I typed this phrase, I had to stop and decide if it was true. Seems like some days, my best hope _is_ found in what doctors say. Although I know in my heart that "to live is Christ and to die is gain" (going to heaven), when death possibly becomes more imminent, it's time to evaluate my choices. Do I _really_ believe that? Have I _really_ placed my trust in the Lord and not in what the medical community can do? I believe I have. Given the opportunity to abandon those decisions of the past based on what I am feeling today, I choose not to undo anything! One of my favorite hymns has this phrase, "My faith has found a resting place." That place is Jesus.

In the early follow-up stages with all my doctors, they seemed happy enough to see me, review the blood work, and in general check how I was doing. In early July 2001 I had a routine mammogram done on my right breast. Dr. Hollen's office called me and said the report came back that the breast tissue was very dense, so an ultrasound was recommended to more clearly see all the tissue. Then I got a letter stating that there "was a finding that needs more study." That upset me more than a little! I was frustrated that the letter arrived on a Saturday and I had to wait until the next Monday to call Dr. Hollen's office. The report stated that there was nothing unusual seen, but given my high risk for breast cancer, they recommended further study using the ultrasound.

I must admit that in those days of waiting I had wrestled with my own thoughts: What if something had been seen? What if the cancer is back? Why so soon? Didn't any of the treatments really work? It would be easy for me to take those thoughts and run with them to the darkest of outcomes. But, the Lord really stepped in and helped me take my thoughts captive and put it in perspective as I waited on the results.

Monday, 16 July

I am afraid. I got a call this morning from Jackie in Dr. Hollen's office. The results of the ultrasound show a "suspicious mass" in the right breast. It's "only" one centimeter. When she was telling me this news I could hardly breathe. As soon as I hung up, I went into the bathroom at work and cried. What else could I do? After a few minutes I thought I had pulled myself together enough to keep working. Some friends were in the office, so I asked them to stop and pray for me. Nona did what a good friend will do—she hugged me tight, cried with me for a while, and then prayed. I am so thankful they were there. Not sure what I would have done alone.

After that I decided an early lunch was in order. I needed to tell James, but how? Go to where he was working? Meet for lunch? I decided to call him. I would prefer not to give this news on the phone, but rather that than in a public place. He was shocked, as I was.

What next? I'm scheduled for an "ultrasound guided core biopsy" on July 24, one week from tomorrow. I hate this waiting. I want to go in tomorrow and have results right away!!!!! Just as life is getting back to normal, there's bad news. Part of me knows it could be just a small cyst or something inconsequential. The bigger part, though, is fearful that cancer has spread and I'll be back in treatment. Or worse—they'll tell me it's untreatable and I have only a certain amount of time to live.

Is it true: "to live is Christ, to die is gain?" Jesus, I want to have faith for the best and to believe that your will is for me to be healed and whole. But I don't know how to have faith like that. Would you give me the faith I need to believe for your best for me? Will you give me assurance that you are with me?

Tuesday, 28 August

Well, a lot has happened. I haven't felt like writing in a while, so I'll try to catch up. The week of waiting for the biopsy was long and unending. Even worse was the waiting between the biopsy being done and the results coming in. Before he did the biopsy, the doctor told me he believed the ultrasound showed no characteristics of a cancerous tumor, but the biopsy would confirm his reading of the mammogram and ultrasound. That put me somewhat at ease, though it was still a difficult few days. He said the results should be in on Wednesday afternoon (after the Tues. morning biopsy), but it was LATE Friday before they called. I called his office on Thursday, only to be told that an "extra test" was being done on the tissue sent in. Naturally, this freaked me out. What kind of test? Why? Was the reading uncertain? Would it come back with a conclusive final report? All of this just about did me in!

The only thing I could do was keep believing God's best for me would prevail. In the few days after my last writing, I had come to a place of having a little bit of faith for a positive report (in this case "positive" means negative-no cancer). I had several conversations with God similar to the story in scripture of the man who cried, "Lord, I believe; help my unbelief!" Each time I had a little more assurance of the outcome. On a scale of 1 to 10, I think I went from a minus 4 to maybe a 2—not able to say "I have faith to be healed" but able to believe God just might want to do something here and now in me. It was more than a "hope so" kind of feeling and I had a lot of ping-pong emotions, but each time, I came back to the place of trust in the Lord.

Late Friday when the nurse called and practically shouted into the phone, IT'S BENIGN, I was speechless— for a moment. She had called my cell phone while I was

driving. Recognizing her number, I pulled on to a side street
and stopped the car. At first, my breathing stopped, and then
of course, the tears started flowing. Even now, as I am writ-
ing, I am crying, moved to tears when I remember.
Indeed, God is good—all the time.

Shortly after this event, James and I went to Eureka Springs,
Arkansas, for a short vacation. It had been some time since we
had been out of town. We rented a cottage and roamed through
lots of antique stores in and around town, walked through part
of downtown, stopped at the Rocky Mountain Chocolate
Factory for a "killer" caramel apple (yummy!). Friday evening
we drove down the road to Inspiration Point, where we saw a
magnificent sunset. Absolutely stunning!

I had returned to a full schedule at work just after the first of
May, though there were many days I was exhausted by the time
I got home. Part of me said to take it easy, be careful not to
over-commit. The other part said that since I was not in treatment, I should be back to my "normal" self. For all my
reputation of being able to say "no" to people, you'd think this
would be easy for me. I did not think I had to prove myself at
work or to friends, so I wasn't sure where this "over driven"
feeling is coming from. Perhaps a sense of losing time that
needs to be made up.

Early in 2004, I had a biopsy of a supraclavicular mass that
had been discovered by a massage therapist. The mass was in the
soft tissue just above the collar bone. It was on the left side —
same side as where I'd had cancer.

Since I would not return to the surgeon who had done my
mastectomy, I asked my oncologist to refer me to another

surgeon. He was very good at explaining all the possibilities before the biopsy, including the fact that it could be metastatic breast cancer. That was not anything I wanted to hear, but I knew he was giving me the whole truth. This surgeon, unlike the other one, had a very personable manner.

One day, between the time I met with the doctor and the biopsy procedure, my dad called. My dad reads through the Bible many times each year, so it did not surprise me at all when he said he had been reading the Old Testament book of Nahum. However, it did catch me off guard when he said there was a word of encouragement for me in the seventh verse of Chapter One. I wrote it down and promised to look it up after work.

Have you ever read the Book of Nahum? There just isn't much encouragement there. It is gloom and doom! With the exception of the first nine verses, all three chapters are about the judgment and wrath of God against a people who have rejected him over and over and over again.

But I read verse 7, *"The Lord is good, a refuge in times of trouble. He cares for those who trust in him."*

That's good! So I kept reading and came to verse 9: *"Whatever they plot against the Lord he will bring to an end; trouble will not come a second time."* This leaped off the page and into my heart! In my mind I cried out, "YES! This is what I want for me right now. I want to believe that this is for me, from God. Cancer is trouble for me and I don't want it to come back a second time." At the time I told no one of this little discovery, not even James. I wanted time to let it germinate before talking about it.

Sure enough, what was at first a fist-pumping "YES!" became a mustard seed of faith that this truly was a word from God for me at just this time. After I shared that with James, my parents, and then some of our friends, it was easy to go in for the biopsy with faith intact, trusting God for the outcome to be good.

When the pathology report came back, I was not surprised that it was benign. The mass was made up of mastectomy scar tissue that had slowly made its way to that point. The only concern I had was the blockage it created in my lymph nodes in that area. That added one more obstacle for the lymph fluid to hurdle in an already compromised area. The surgeon was careful to remove what he could without creating even more scar tissue in the area.

I don't want to ever forget what God did for me that day, February 27, 2004, when he spoke a word and faith was born. This faith was not salvation-faith or faith that God could/might do something, but faith that he *would* do something on my behalf. It's worth remembering!

There was another scare in May 2005. Since I had been coughing for a few days my family doctor decided to take a chest x-ray to rule out pneumonia. He sent me home by way of my pharmacy with instructions to take the week off and get some rest. (I love this doctor!)

Two days later he called to see how I was doing. My surprise at his call turned to apprehension when he hesitated and then said, "Annette, I see a small shadow on your x-ray and I'm concerned about it." I remember that I was reaching for something and my hand just stopped in mid-air. He then told me that he wanted me to see my oncologist immediately and he would have them call me for an appointment.

I was devastated! I called James immediately and told him the news. It was late in the afternoon so I knew I could only wait for Dr. Hollen's office to call. Early the next day I heard from his nurse. Two tests were scheduled, to be completed before I would meet with Dr. Hollen to review the results.

I called or e-mailed everyone I could think of to ask them to pray for me. I was so scared and just knew inside of me that this couldn't be good. It would be the following week before the whole-body CT and PET scans could be done, so there I was again—waiting, waiting, waiting.

The CT scan is intended to analyze bone structure. The newer, more expensive PET scan looks for unusual activity in the soft tissue. For the PET scan, glucose was injected intravenously so the scan could pick up any "hot spots" of activity. Cancer cells are known to use up more glucose than normal cells, so when there is a cluster of cancer cells, it shows up on the PET scan.

The tests were done and then the mandatory waiting period was endured. When James and I met with Dr. Hollen he immediately told us there was no sign of cancer! My tests were so normal, they were called "boring." You can call me boring any day when you tell me I don't have cancer!

So what caused the shadow on the x-ray? Apparently during radiation treatment, the very top of the left lobe of the lung was damaged just enough to cause my diaphragm to be slightly elevated. That elevation caused the shadow and also explained why I am frequently out of breath. (Being aerobically out of shape wouldn't have anything to do with that, of course!)

My personality is such that I would love to mark an "A" beside each one of these faith-building opportunities and call them done. In reality, life doesn't work that way. Life takes us on a journey, winding this way and that. Where we end up depends on where our roots are. God gave me a word picture to help me remember that life is a process.

Several years ago, James and I were driving back home from west Texas. We had been visiting with our sisters—mine in Plainview, his in Lubbock. We were driving north on the very straight, very boring Interstate 27. James was driving while I looked at the scenery, such as it was in west Texas in the winter. I have a very fertile imagination and like to get lost in my thoughts about what an area would have been like before roads were cut in, before towns and cities scattered the landscape. Off to the west side of the road, set in the middle of a dormant cotton field, was a very large tree. There aren't many large trees in that part of the country and this lone giant caught my attention. I studied it for the few minutes it was in sight—a huge tree in the arid countryside, so I knew the roots went deep. The branches were wide and barren of leaves, revealing all the twists and turns as they made their way skyward.

The most striking thing about the tree was how the branches all seemed to lean northward. In an instant, I knew why. In this part of the country, the prevailing wind is from the south. Anything that is outside—flags, clothes on the line, trash, even trees—will be blowing northward soon.

God spoke to me through that tree. You see, life is like a blowing wind. We are all going to be blown around some, first this way and then that way. Happy moments and joyful blessings get us going one direction, only to get yanked around by an illness, a financial catastrophe, or some other unwanted life event. But what holds us in place? Where are our roots ... those deeply-held beliefs that keep us grounded?

I have chosen to keep my roots planted in my faith in God. Just like that west Texas tree, I want to be strong enough at my foundation that I go only in the direction where the wind of

God takes me. A relationship with Jesus is not a mystical, strange phenomenon. The mystery is that God loves me just as I am! What I understand even more today than ever before is that God wants to grow me up from an immature sapling into a strong spiritual tree to reflect His beauty, grace and strength.

One of my favorite blessings in all of scripture is Ephesians 3:16-21:

> *"I pray that out of his glorious riches he may strengthen you with power through his Spirit in your inner being, so that Christ may dwell in your hearts through faith. And I pray that you, being rooted and established in love, may have power, together with all the saints, to grasp how wide and long and high and deep is the love of Christ, and to know this love that surpasses knowledge – that you may be filled to the measure of all the fullness of God.*
>
> *"Now to him who is able to do immeasurably more than all we ask or imagine, according to his power that is at work within us, to him be glory in the church and in Christ Jesus throughout all generations, for ever and ever! Amen."*

I am learning that God's love for me is strong enough to carry me through anything a new day can bring. Whenever I wear my pink awareness ribbon I am reminded of the faith walk through cancer that started a few years ago. My cancer is in remission but there are new challenges in the world. Loved ones pass away. Financial hardship is common. Uncertainty abounds.

So, whatever you're facing today ... whatever awareness ribbon represents your situation ... I hope that you, too, will allow it to be a ribbon of faith!